Measuring the Impact of Dyslexia

Measuring the Impact of Dyslexia shows the considerable benefits of recognising and celebrating the skills of those with information processing differences, explains their unique brain organisation and shows how they can excel as contributing members of society with proper support and guidance. It offers a balanced and research-based perspective to living with this condition, highlighting the huge number of children leaving school with low literacy levels, as a result of undiagnosed information processing differences.

Full of critically reflective questions, case studies and interviews with those affected by dyslexia, this text encourages educators of children and young people with dyslexia to challenge their own perceptions by understanding the links between low literacy and anti-social behaviour, poor health, unemployment and limited educational attainment, and includes helpful pointers for improving practice and outcomes.

This accessible and readable text is aimed at students, practitioners, researchers and experienced professionals in a range of disciplines to enhance CPD. It is particularly relevant for students working on both taught and research based masters degrees, especially programmes related to specific learning difficulties.

Carol Hayes most recently held the position of Principal Lecturer in Early Childhood Studies at Staffordshire University; she is a visiting lecturer for Weston University Centre (Bath Spa University) and is an external examiner for the Open University.

Measuring the Impact of Dyslexia

Striking a Successful Balance for Individuals, Families and Society

Carol Hayes

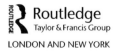
LONDON AND NEW YORK

First published 2021
by Routledge
2 Park Square, Milton Park, Abingdon, Oxon OX14 4RN

and by Routledge
52 Vanderbilt Avenue, New York, NY 10017

Routledge is an imprint of the Taylor & Francis Group, an informa business

© 2021 Carol Hayes

The right of Carol Hayes to be identified as author of this work has been asserted by her in accordance with sections 77 and 78 of the Copyright, Designs and Patents Act 1988.

All rights reserved. No part of this book may be reprinted or reproduced or utilised in any form or by any electronic, mechanical, or other means, now known or hereafter invented, including photocopying and recording, or in any information storage or retrieval system, without permission in writing from the publishers.

Trademark notice: Product or corporate names may be trademarks or registered trademarks, and are used only for identification and explanation without intent to infringe.

British Library Cataloguing-in-Publication Data
A catalogue record for this book is available from the British Library

Library of Congress Cataloging-in-Publication Data
Names: Hayes, Carol (Lecturer in early childhood studies) author.
Title: Measuring the impact of dyslexia : striking a successful balance for individuals, families and society / Carol Hayes.
Description: Abingdon, Oxon ; New York, NY : Routledge, 2020. | Includes bibliographical references and index.
Identifiers: LCCN 2020008583 (print) | LCCN 2020008584 (ebook) | ISBN 9780367195366 (hardback) | ISBN 9780367195380 (paperback) | ISBN 9780429203008 (ebook)
Subjects: LCSH: Dyslexia. | Dyslexia--Social aspects. | Dyslexics--Rehabilitation.
Classification: LCC RC394.W6 H39 2020 (print) | LCC RC394.W6 (ebook) | DDC 616.85/53--dc23
LC record available at https://lccn.loc.gov/2020008583
LC ebook record available at https://lccn.loc.gov/2020008584

ISBN: 978-0-367-19536-6 (hbk)
ISBN: 978-0-367-19538-0 (pbk)
ISBN: 978-0-429-20300-8 (ebk)

Typeset in Bembo
by Taylor & Francis Books

Contents

List of illustrations — vi
Foreword — vii
Acknowledgements — xi
Glossary — xii

1. Introduction to dyslexia — 1
2. Help! I'm drowning! — 22
3. The cost to family and friends — 40
4. Health and mental health — 57
5. The cost to education and social service — 74
6. The criminal justice system — 93
7. Employment: Cost to employers/employees — 110
8. Balancing the books: Advantages to society — 126
9. Research and academia — 144
10. The great dyslexia industry — 158
11. Politics, politics and policy — 177

    Endnote — 191

    Index — 192

Illustrations

Figures

1.1	All the same but very different	6
1.2	Adaptation of the Johari window	7
2.1	Self-esteem and the ideal self	27
2.2	The hierarchy of self-esteem	27
2.3	Cycle of success and high self-esteem	31
2.4	The growth mindset	33
4.1	Cyclical process of criticism leading to depression	59
4.2	Graduated scale of depression	63
4.3	Mind map	67
5.1	Variables to inclusive practice	81
5.2	Results of small-scale survey of social work students (2018)	88
5.3	Small-scale survey of thirty-four social work students' understanding of dyslexia	90
6.1	Cycle of anti-social behaviour and criminality	95
6.2	The cycle of failure	104
8.1	Hemispheres of the brain (diagram first published in Hayes, 2019)	133
8.2	Brain structure (diagram first published in Hayes, 2019)	134
8.3	Normal distribution curve for axons	135
8.4	Dyslexia support	138
8.5	Redefining success	140
9.1	Brief history of the understanding of the brain	146
9.2	Bridging the chasm from researchers to practitioners	152
11.1	Collaboration and the interrelationship with dyslexia	184

Tables

1.1	The historical context of dyslexia	3
7.1	Common difficulties in the workplace	113
8.1	Some of the talents attributed to dyslexia	129
9.1	Types of research	151
10.1	Evaluating the overall strength of the evidence	163

Foreword

Carol Hayes worked in early years for over 40 years as a deputy head teacher, teacher and tutor. I first met her at Staffordshire University where she was principal lecturer and academic group leader where she helped to develop the early childhood studies department with programmes from Foundation Degrees to Masters. Until recently she was the National Chair for the Sector Endorsed Foundation Degrees in Early Years Professional Association (SEFDEY), where she was an integral part of the development of this association, working tirelessly to enhance the academic profile of early years. Those earliest learning opportunities are slowly being recognised as the most vital time for the education and care of young children; Carol has championed this cause since the 1970s.

When I was asked to write this foreword for Carol, I felt it was an enormous task and sat in front of a screen wondering how I could find a way to express my gratitude with respect to the author, for the impact she has had on not only my life but that of many others. I hope through this introduction to the author and her work you too feel the dedication and passion this lady has for better outcomes for children, through raising practitioner knowledge, understanding and self-worth.

I met Carol in January 2008 when I was finishing my BA (Hons) in early childhood studies, at Staffordshire University. I was lucky enough to be doing this at the height of the graduate leader funding in England, when early years degrees had been designed to enhance the qualification and pedagogy of practitioners, based on new research and understanding of how children learn. We have often laughed about our first meeting, when Carol spoke to the class, introducing herself as a lady with high expectations for this new leading role which we were creating within early years. I came away feeling scared and overwhelmed with the responsibility that had been placed on my shoulders. I soon began to realise that below an authoritative exterior, it was this desire to raise the quality and standards within early years and to gain the recognition for our work that was at the heart of Carol's passion. Equally the look Carol had when she gave me a mark for an assignment brought tears to my eyes, and we both realised she believed in me more than I did myself.

From our very first meeting Carol has inspired me in my work as a practitioner, and later a university lecturer. She encouraged me to raise my aspirations, developing my own beliefs and understanding around research linked directly to my practice, and taking that forward to help me understand my own impact on others. This allowed me to see life experiences as a positive influence on my practice, thereby embracing opportunities to raise my own academic and professional status.

Carol encouraged and believed in my journey as a student and supported me through the BA (Hons) and throughout the Master's degree that followed. Once completed, we became friends, Carol has often been my critical friend in my professional life, supporting me through conversations and debates to question the education system of the future. Carol has encouraged me to make a move in my older years from practice to a lecturer at Coventry University, where I can continue to pass on the passion that was gifted to me.

It was Carol who introduced me to the underpinning knowledge around dyslexia; like Carol, I too have dyslexia in the family, but had been led to understand this learning difference as a disability. Indeed, you will often find us in a garden centre coffee shop deconstructing the phenomenology of dyslexia. Carol wrote her PhD on dyslexia: "Policy and Prevalence of Dyslexia in Wales". Where Dr Hayes concluded that although support for dyslexia is progressive with the growing support of policy, there is still a need to improve the pedagogy and public understanding of dyslexia, forming a collaboration between health, education and economic policy. The widening educational inequalities can breed many social problems for children and continue later as adults. However, evidence suggests that investing in their future will help to form competent and aspirational adults.

As retirement loomed Carol was not yet ready to pass over the baton for fighting the early years fight with a focus on dyslexia. Carol began to write books that she felt were needed within the profession. Carol's writing has further added to her journey, clearly defining her thought process as she negotiates the complicated minefield that education in early years has become. For me it is Carol's writing style that makes her books so interesting; she provides an easily digestible, accessible yet critical approach within early years research, using key themes to help the reader make direct links to practice and their own personal beliefs. Almost like peeling an onion, Carol unveils through her work, layer by layer, to explore deeper the underpinning understanding to supporting children in their language processing and assimilation. Carol opened her book writing journey with the book *Developing as a Reflective Early Years Practitioner* (C. Hayes et al., 2014; 2nd edn 2017), exploring the surface of the onion, written with her colleagues of the time. Through examining the impact of reflection on practice, the authors considered how reflecting on improving practice could produce a more responsive and thoughtful, research-based workforce, for young children and their families.

Her second book and first on her own, *Language, Literacy and Communication in the Early Years: A Critical Foundation* (2016), explores the importance of those early interactions, thus peeling back to the fleshy part of the onion, determining the holistic nature of child development. Carol again ensured that knowledge and research was presented in workable amounts to reach practitioners effectively. She continues to examine a deficit medical view of children with communication difficulties that can lead to a risk of poor outcomes educationally, socially and in employment. Using theories and research into the acquisition of young children's language and literacy, she considers a range of interventions that depend on practitioner understanding and effective delivery. Carol uses pedagogical features that encourage a questioning, challenging and reflective approach, promoting critical thinking throughout.

The book *Developmental Dyslexia from Birth to Eight* (2018) precedes her current writing and introduces her true passion in supporting children with dyslexia to access the earliest and most effective intervention available. Contrary to previous discussions around the medical deficit model of dyslexia, Carol explores an innovative approach that considers the modern neurological advances that investigate the diverse nature of dyslexia. When referring to the onion, it is clear that the heart of the issue is approached, but as with many of these neurological conditions there are often more than one heart to the onion, with considerations of the variables that impact on a child's learning throughout their life. The book outlines the pivotal role practitioners play in supporting and encouraging children with dyslexia; by understanding the condition to a deeper level, from the origins and identification of dyslexia, through to national and global policy on provision for children with dyslexia, practitioners are empowered through the adaptation of pedagogy.

Finally, I come to this book. I feel honoured to have read the advance copy, which I do not hesitate in saying is Dr Hayes' best book so far. At the beginning of this I wondered how I could provide a fitting tribute that expressed my gratitude for all my friend has done for me over the years. I feel this has enabled me to fulfil that desire so thank you Dr Hayes for everything. Throughout this book Carol cleverly engages in a collection of retrospective interviews with dyslexic adults, encouraging them to reflect on their journey together with their relationship with the condition. She then uses the theory and research to contemplate the level of support and intervention these adults have received, leading to the long-term impact throughout the life of a dyslexic adult. The interviews consider aspirations, diagnosis, resilience, education and strengths. The shocking statistics relating to the criminal justice system can no longer be ignored. I was particularly interested in the learned helplessness, parental denial and mental health impacts that are directly linked to the diagnosis or experience of dyslexia. Carol clearly outlines the long-term impacts of a deficit model and explores the positives of a shift in the perception of dyslexia. From her early thesis into dyslexia, Carol recognised that there is still a need to improve the pedagogy and public understanding of dyslexia, forming a collaboration between health, education and economic policy, to reduce the widening educational inequalities. Through her writing Carol continues this very important fight.

Dr Hayes' innovative approach to dyslexia values the emerging neuroscience and how this knowledge could lead a wind of change for the perception of the condition, a line of thought I personally would like to follow. It is clearly identified by the participants that the most challenging barriers associated with the condition are their experiences during their educational journey. There is a growing recognition within the leading global employment platform, which relies on creativity and curiosity to value the dyslexic skills. With increased training and understanding, teachers can be given the skills to adapt their teaching to the world of a dyslexic child; this in turn could hopefully change aspiration and outcomes to celebrate the advantages dyslexic MIND strengths have for our society.

An engaging, accessible and fascinating insight into truly understanding dyslexia, this book is written in a clear and informative way that would be an advantage to not only practitioners, but equally to families who live with dyslexia on a day-to-day basis. As my friend and continued mentor, Carol has inspired my own PhD mission, which will focus on the dyslexic journey. If we are really committed to changing a system that struggles to support dyslexic children, then this book should be placed in every setting to support our pedagogy for the future.

Debbie Nye
Senior Lecturer Early Years Coventry University

Acknowledgements

My heartfelt thanks to all who have contributed freely to this book; without those who have, on occasions, poured out their heart to me, reliving often painful experiences of their life with dyslexia, this book could not have been written. All interviewees were anonymised, but gave their time and attention to this book, to help to advance the knowledge and support that should be readily available to those with dyslexia, but, as most of them have attested to, has not always been available in the past.

My thanks also to Lewis Hayes for his illustrations which have enriched the text and made the book more readable and comprehensible. It is because of the struggles that I witnessed in Lewis that this book was written at all.

Thank you also to Barry for his invaluable technical support.

My grateful thanks as ever, for my long-suffering husband, who has been a 'book widower' for the last two years!

Glossary

declarative learning   Learning that can be talked about, learning about things like historical facts and information. This is the way to construct meaning and organise and store knowledge, rather than procedural learning which is learning the steps or skills of a manual activity, such as mending a bike.

demand characteristics   Signals which a researcher may unconsciously transmit to a participant in their research which may indicate how they expect them to behave or respond.

diffusion tensor imaging (DTI)   An imaging technique for identifying microstructural changes in the central nervous system by measuring the diffusion of water molecules within brain tissue.

Education, Health and Care (EHC) plan   A plan devised for children and young people aged up to 25 years who need additional support for their special needs. It may provide access to additional funding to support those needs, whether they are educational, health or social care related.

electroencephalography (EEG)   This measures and records the electrical activity in the brain, by attaching sensors externally to the scalp. Abnormal activity can be interpreted by a specially trained neurophysiologist.

equifinality   An end point can be achieved from a range of different directions. Two children with vastly different backgrounds and early experiences can still end up achieving at the same level.

functional magnetic resonance imaging (fMRI)   A technique to measure neuronal activity. Areas of the brain that are active require more oxygen to work effectively; this requires an increase in blood flow. The fMRI measures the blood flow to parts of the brain; it is safe to use and non-invasive.

informed consent   This is essential to ethical research. Each participant is allowed access to information about the research, what it is and what it will be used for. They are under no pressure to participate and may need time to consider the implications for them of taking part. This would normally be in writing and, when the participant is fully aware of all the facts and asked all their questions, they will be asked to sign to say that they understand. No pressure should be put on anyone to participate and they must be aware that at any point in the research they can withdraw without having to give detailed explanations.

magnetic resonance imaging (MRI)   This uses strong magnetic fields and radio waves to scan soft tissues of the body to 3D images. It is painless and safe, if a little uncomfortable, as the subject is required to lie motionless as they are moved through a large tube. Some people have described this as like having your head in the washing machine!

magnetic resonance spectroscopy (MRS)   Also known as NMR (nuclear magnetic resonance). This is non-invasive and allows a researcher to see biochemical processes as they occur in the body. MRS can be used on body fluids, cell extracts and tissue samples.

magnetoencephalography (MEG)   This is used to review the electrical activity in the brain between neurons. It is highly sensitive and can detect minute magnetic fields.

phonographic system of writing   A writing system that relies on the sounds that make up words.

positron emission tomography (PET)   A small amount of radioactive material is inserted into the body and can measure physiological function by looking at blood flow, metabolism, neurotransmitters and radiolabelled drugs.

real time communication (RTC)   Instant electronic exchange of information/communication.

savant syndrome   A rare condition whereby a person whose intellectual abilities are to or below norm exhibits, remarkable cognitive gifts such as mathematical calculations, memory feats, musical talents, etc.

zone of proximal development (ZPD)   A term coined by the Soviet psychologist Lev Vygotsky that refers to the gap between what a person can learn on their own through their own discovery, and what they can learn through the guidance of a teacher or peer with a higher skill set.

1 Introduction to dyslexia

> No one who can read, ever looks at a book, even 'unopened on a shelf' like the one who cannot.
> Dickens (1998, p. 22; original publication 1865)

Introduction

I wanted to write this book to highlight the impact that dyslexia can have, both positive and negative, upon individuals, families, employers, employment chances, education, the health service, the criminal justice system and society in general. I fully recognise that there are potentially many positive consequences for society and we could all probably benefit more by valuing those who think differently, those who are able to think 'outside the box' and perceive the world from divergent perspectives.

The book is aimed at all those who are planning to work professionally with adults and children who are dyslexic and those in training, but also for those who are just interested in this fascinating area of cognitive research. I hope that I will show that although dyslexia should rightly be a cause for general public concern, if appropriately valued, it could also make a positive contribution to employment and the economy through entrepreneurship and innovation

The book aims to analyse the impact upon society and the individual and to challenge the perception that because of the large numbers who could potentially be identified with dyslexia, we cannot afford to put suitable support in place. In our highly computerised and technically sophisticated world we have more and more to learn and literacy has become essential, as most learning ultimately requires reading. Modern society can be badly impacted when literacy cannot be relied upon.

Dyslexia in context

It is important for your understanding that dyslexia is set within the context of a historical framework. This will enable you to understand how recently this condition has been identified, and the range of occupations and professions that have been involved with that identification. Dyslexia has been on a difficult historical journey, going as far back as the 1800s when a few people could see that this was a condition which required investigation.

In the 1960s to 1980s the whole concept of dyslexia was derided by many as educational mumbo-jumbo. Dyslexia was frequently referred to as the middle-class disease, with the idea that educated middle-class parents needed an excuse for why their child was not reading. Frequently they felt that the blame fell upon them for not reading to and with their children, or not giving them enough of their time. Guilt was often very high. Today it is probably rare to find anyone who does not accept that there is a condition (whatever it may be called) that is neurological and probably genetic in origin, which makes it difficult for affected individuals to process information in the way that others do. Whether this condition can be clearly defined by the experts or not, it does exist, making the problem not with the affected individual but rather with the experts who are unable to agree. In order to understand the historical line that this condition has taken I have put the significant moments into Table 1.1; the table also identifies the many different professions which have become involved with the identification and progression of the condition.

Definition

The origin of the word 'dyslexia' is probably Greek, with 'dys' meaning bad, ill or difficult (as in dyspepsia, dysentery and dystopia) and 'lexia' which refers to words (as in lexicographer, lexicon, etc). In one sentence dyslexia has become known as someone who has difficulty with words. This is certainly the traditional definition and some small-scale research which I conducted for my last book (Hayes, 2018) showed that when asked what dyslexia was, most people in the survey of the general population said that it related to a difficulty with literacy. However, if dyslexia is only about reading and literacy delay then all children who struggle with reading would be described as dyslexic. Today the word dyslexia is certainly used by non-specialists in common parlance, and most people believe that they know what it means, but at one time it was a specialist medical term only used in the medical profession. Researchers such as Cutting et al. (2013) suggest that the neurobiology of those with dyslexia is very different to those with other reading difficulties such as specific reading comprehension deficit (S-RCD). These differences can be seen in aetiology, genetics, cognition, neurobiology and developmentally, setting those with dyslexia apart from those with general learning difficulties and those with other specific reading difficulties.

It has been almost a century and a quarter since this condition was first observed, and in 1896 it was described in a British Medical Journal as a visual processing difficulty (Morgan, 1896). However, research has moved on and indicates that dyslexia is probably so much more than simply a difficulty with literacy; using the single term dyslexia rather implies that it is a single condition with a known neurological origin, but over the years researchers such as

Table 1.1 The historical context of dyslexia

Date	Historic event	Occupation
877	Adolph Kussmaul Identified a condition that he called 'word blindness'.	Neurologist
1887	Rudolph Berlin Coined the word 'dyslexia'.	Ophthalmologist
1896	William Pringle-Morgan Published the paper 'A Case of Congenital Word Blindness'.	British physician
1917	James Hinshelwood Wrote about a case study of Percy F, a bright 14-year-old with literacy difficulties.	Eye surgeon
1926	Samuel Orton Set up the first training under the Orton Society.	American psychiatrist
1962	Kenneth Thompson Made the first mention of dyslexia in Parliament.	Member of Parliament
1964	MacDonald Critchley Published the seminal book Developmental Dyslexia; later in 1970 this was updated to The Dyslexic Child.	Neurologist
1970	Lord Morris of Manchester (Alf Morris) Introduced the 'The Chronically Sick and Disabled Persons Act' which mentions dyslexia as a disability for the first time in law.	Member of Parliament
1972	The British Dyslexia Association was formed.	Voluntary organisation
1975	Sir Alan Bullock Produced the Bullock Report (A Language for Life) and recommended specialist support for children with dyslexia.	Vice Chancellor, Oxford University
1977	Professor Tim Miles Set up the Bangor Dyslexia Unit at Bangor University, North Wales.	Professor Emeritus of Psychology, Bangor University

(*Continued*)

Table 1.1 (Cont.)

Date	Historic event	Occupation
1987	The Government finally recognises dyslexia as a disability.	The Hansard records the Commons sitting where this is discussed by The Right Hon. David Amess MP
1994	The Dyslexia Guild is formed This is a professional organisation for all those working professionally with dyslexia to help them to improve the support that they offer.	
2009	Sir Jim Rose Published Identifying and Teaching Children and Young People with Dyslexia and Literacy Difficulties (known as the Rose Review).	Her Majesty's Chief Inspector (HMI) of Primary Education, and Director of Inspection for the Office for Standards in Education (OFSTED) in England
2010	The Equality Act Protects people with dyslexia in the workplace. Employers must make reasonable adjustments.	HM Government UK
2016	A Starbucks employee with dyslexia wins a disability discrimination case.	Legal profession

Frith (1997) and Miles (2001) have shown that defining dyslexia as one entity is unhelpful and probably misleading. More likely it is a combination of many different kinds of brain working and development that interact with the environmental conditions they are exposed to. This is one reason why I would rather refer to dyslexia as part of an information processing difference (IPD), which has the potential to influence the holistic development of the person and be recognisable in a combination of physical, memory, cognitive and language differences, often resulting in profound and life-changing social and emotional difficulties.

It is generally agreed that dyslexia is a condition on the autistic spectrum, which is rarely, if ever, seen without a combination of co-morbid conditions such as developmental coordination disorder (dyspraxia), dyscalculia, attention deficit and hyperactivity disorder, specific language disorder, Asperger's and many others. This is another reason why I prefer to talk about an IPD, which enables a more global and differentiated view of how people experience this condition. Discussing dyslexia in this manner does have considerable advantages for securing a definition, and probably leads the lay person to a better understanding of a complex, multifaceted condition and the relationship between dyslexia (a condition usually related to words and literacy) and the other observable behaviours that people with this condition often exhibit. This then makes sense to the individual with dyslexia, and those close to them, who struggle to understand what they are feeling and why. This concept of difference in the way that the brain processes information that it receives (whether related to literacy or not) will be assumed throughout this book. It is vital for an understanding of this multidimensional condition that it is seen under a broader perspective, not limited to reading or spelling or even confined to literacy and language skills, rather that these are merely symptomatic and are probably the most observable of a much broader and pervasive difference of information processing. Poor literacy skills alone cannot constitute a definition, but are merely one aspect of the issue, and not necessarily even a crucial or exclusive one.

Although an IPD is so much more than a difficulty with words, for many this is the most observable and measurable feature for identification. However, it is also true that most people with dyslexia *can* read and, in some cases, they read well; this is attested to by the number of students in higher education with IPDs. The HESA (Higher Education Statistics Agency) data for 2016–2017 reveals that more than 22,000 students with Specific Learning Difficulties (SpLD) were in higher education in the UK (HESA, 2017), but for many the issue is not being unable to identify the words on a page, but the speed of processing, making them slow to read and comprehend. Anyone who has listened to a new young reader will be aware of how having to concentrate so hard on each presenting word can mean a loss of comprehension. Sit with many four- and five-year-olds and after they have struggled to get to the end of a passage, they will often be completely unable to tell you what they have read. Each word was correctly pronounced and identified, but no meaning was attached to the overall sentence and the 'reading' becomes slow and monotonal.

The overwhelming difficulty with identifying this condition is that those with IPDs do not look different or sound different to anyone else; looking at any group of people it is unlikely to be possible to recognise which ones have IPDs and which do not. It is like looking at a line of terraced houses; on first glance they all appear to be very similar and there is no way to see what is happening inside (Figure 1.1).

However, inside each house it is very different, with relationships going on, arguments, turmoil, emotions, different furniture, different decoration and structures, order and disorder, all hidden from view, but each will significantly influence those who live within them. In this respect the model of the Johari window (Figure 1.2) may be useful to understand this.

Similarly, Nosek (1997) talks about differing awareness and disclosure of dyslexia, with three different types of person with the condition:

- The *candid dyslexic*: the individual is fully aware of their learning differences and is willing to reveal this to others.
- The *closet dyslexic*: the individual is aware but attempts to conceal it, sometimes even from themselves, in misplaced shame and fear.
- The *confused dyslexic*: the individual is unaware of their dyslexia and struggles through life and education not knowing why they have such difficulty compared to their peers.

Developmental dyslexia is almost certainly heritable and genetically transmitted in an autosomal dominant pattern, that is, you only need to have one parent with the gene or gene cluster to inherit that condition. It is also

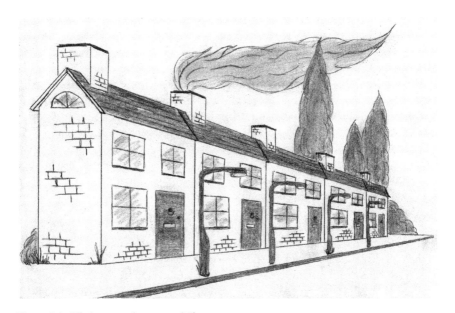

Figure 1.1 All the same but very different

Introduction to dyslexia 7

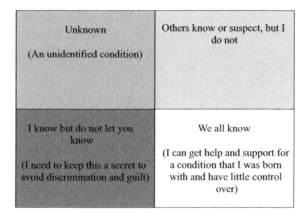

Figure 1.2 Adaptation of the Johari window
Adapted from Luft and Ingham (1955)

associated with neuroanatomical anomalies such as a reduced volume of grey matter in parts of the brain and reduced regional white matter in other parts, compared with non-dyslexic individuals (Xia et al., 2016). If a distinct genetic condition does exist then it must be completely unconnected to an individual's life experience, attitudes to and opinions of education, the home learning environment, culture, socio-economics, personality and, crucially, unrelated to the way in which they are taught. However, that is not to say that differences in all of these and other environmental influences cannot influence the way that a person experiences and manages their IPD and how they develop their strengths and abilities.

Reid (2016) emphasises how important a definition can be and indicates many reasons why eventually we have to arrive at a mutually accepted definition. A definition is essential for:

- The allocation of support and resources
- Providing an explanation and understanding for teachers and professionals
- Enabling better understanding for parents and families
- Enabling better self-knowledge for the individual, and eventually helping them to develop coping mechanisms
- Enabling the individual to focus upon their strengths
- Informing the nature of appropriate and targeted intervention
- Enabling reliable and valid research, as well-defined samples can be used for detailed further enquiry.

Many have tried to develop a definition, but this alone probably adds to the confusion as they all want to put their own nuanced stamp upon it. Probably the most used and referred to definition is promoted by the British Dyslexia Association, which defines the condition as:

8 Introduction to dyslexia

> A specific learning difficulty which mainly affects the development of literacy and language related skills. It is likely to be present at birth and is lifelong in its effects. It is characterised by difficulties with phonological processing, rapid naming, working memory, processing speed and the automatic development of skills that may not match up to an individual's other cognitive abilities. It tends to be resistant to conventional teaching methods, but its effects can be mitigated by appropriately specific intervention, including the application of information technology and supportive counselling.
>
> (British Dyslexia Association, 2017)

Although this definition does mention different aspects of the condition, such as *automatic development of skills*, it still largely focuses on reading and skills directly related to literacy.

In 2009 Sir Jim Rose produced, for the government of the day, what is now referred to as the Rose Review. Rose describes dyslexia as:

> A learning difficulty that primarily affects the skills involved in accurate and fluent word reading and spelling.
>
> Characteristic features of dyslexia difficulties in phonological awareness, verbal memory and verbal processing speed.
>
> Dyslexia occurs across the range of intellectual abilities.
>
> It is best thought of as a continuum not a distinct category and there are no clear cut-off points.
>
> Co-occurring difficulties may be seen in aspects of language, motor coordination, mental calculation, concentration and personal organisation but these are not by themselves markers of dyslexia.
>
> (Rose, 2009, p. 10)

The British Psychological Society (BPS) offers the following definition, which has not been radically updated since its inception in 1999:

> Dyslexia is evident when accurate and fluent word reading and/or spelling develops very incompletely or with great difficulty. The problem is severe despite appropriate learning opportunities ... This is learning opportunities that are effective for the great majority of children.
>
> (British Psychological Society, 1999)

This offers a very negative view of the condition, with words such as 'difficulty', 'problem' and 'incomplete' appearing prominently and once again only really relating to reading and literacy. There is no mention of any possible strengths or advantages of the condition.

The International Dyslexia Association (IDA) offers a further definition:

Dyslexia is a specific learning disability that is neurological in origin. It is characterised by difficulties with accurate and/or fluent word recognition and by poor spelling and decoding abilities. These difficulties typically result from a deficit in the phonological component of language that is often unexpected in relation to other cognitive abilities and the provision of effective classroom instruction. Secondary consequences may include problems in reading comprehension and reduced reading experience that can impede the growth of vocabulary and background knowledge.

(International Dyslexia Association, 2002)

Clearly this is also a definition which emphasises the deficits of dyslexia with words such as 'difficulties', 'disability', 'poor', 'problems', 'reduced' and 'impede' featuring highly. Both the BDA (2017) and the IDA (2002) mention a discrepancy between cognitive abilities and expected performance, which is a largely outdated consideration, with most experts in agreement that dyslexia and IPDs can be present in children across the whole spectrum of cognitive ability. Clearly if a child has general learning difficulties professionals may not be expecting them to learn to read; as a consequence their dyslexia, which may be there, may be disguised and therefore overlooked.

A more inclusive definition is given by Reid (2016) who is very experienced in the field, being both a teacher and a psychologist, and shows some similarities, but also some differences, but is still a largely negative definition:

Dyslexia is a processing difference, often characterised by difficulties in literacy acquisition affecting reading, writing and spelling. It can also have an impact on cognitive processes such as memory, speed of processing, time management, coordination and automaticity. Then maybe visual and/or phonological difficulties and there are usually some discrepancies in educational performance.

(Reid, 2016, p. 5)

Without wanting to add to the confusion of definitions, for the purposes of this book I have used the following very open description, to ensure consistency of a more inclusive and less negative approach throughout the text.

Developmental dyslexia is a multifaceted, neurobiological information processing difference potentially affecting the holistic development of the individual, both positively and negatively, from the moment of conception. It may require a more imaginative pedagogy to ensure that each individual reaches their inherent potential.

(Hayes, 2018, p. 13)

It could be that definitions that only focus on literacy and reading are excluding those who, whilst perfectly able to read, still experience problems with personal organisation, mathematics and numerical notation, sequencing, memory, comprehension, physical and motor coordination. It should also be noted that all these definitions focus on a descriptive explanation for dyslexia and do not attempt a causal explanation.

Elliott and Grigorenko (2014) point out that there are very real difficulties with arriving at an agreed definition:

> One of the key difficulties of those who have tried to produce a definition of dyslexia concerns the extent of its inclusivity. Even relatively general definitions have been criticised as too inclusive by some groups and too exclusive by others.
>
> (Elliott and Grigorenko, 2014, p. 8)

One of the problems with some of the more vague definitions offered in the literature is that they are not really addressing the issue from either perspective, and often fail to distinguish between those who are generally poor readers and those who are dyslexic and can have a range of other difficulties not directly related to literacy.

Another difficulty of coming to an agreed definition is that the act of reading itself is so complex and difficult to define. You see someone sitting down with a book open on their lap, they are looking at a book and we make the assumption that they are reading, but this may not be the case. The Shorter Oxford Dictionary occupies nearly two thousand words to describe the act of reading! Reading is an act that we cannot *see* happening, we can only make assumptions about it from the external triggers that we can observe. There are also so many different types of reading:

- Reading aloud
- Reading silently
- Reading a newspaper
- Reading a comic
- Reading a list
- Reading a dictionary
- Reading a novel
- Reading a textbook
- Reading from a screen
- Scanning
- Skimming
- Reading the meter
- Close reading
- Proof reading
- Reading a timetable or calendar
- Predicting and inferring.

These are probably only a few of the many interpretations of the word 'reading', and each one requires different skills and different techniques to be learned for comprehension. There are also the times when we have 'read' a whole page of script only to realise that what we have apparently read has no comprehension, often from fatigue or lack of interest. So, as dyslexia cannot be seen as one entity so the term 'reading' can also be seen as multi-faceted and multi-factorial, which contributes to the reason why developmental dyslexia is so hard to define as a condition. It is far easier to consider it as a wide range of holistic and developmental disturbances of function which are constitutional in origin.

> It seems reasonable … to take a wider perspective than is normal in studies of dyslexia, and to investigate the hypothesis that the nature of the 'dyslexia deficit' is not limited to reading and that the 'dyslexia reading deficit' is merely a symptom of a more general and pervasive deficit in the acquisition of skill.
> (Nicolson and Fawcett, 1990, p. 160)

Tonnessen (1997) suggests that rather than wasting effort searching for an agreed definition of dyslexia, what is needed is a hypothesis, which can be rejected or adapted as new research is forthcoming.

Just as there is no agreed definition of dyslexia or even of reading itself, so there is no agreement about the best way to *teach* reading. Miller (2015) refers to this as 'the Emperor's new clothes', some form of unconscious collusion between teachers, training institutions, government etc., to make parents believe that schools and teachers know the best way to teach their children to read.

> There is no accepted, proven, evidence-based method for teaching reading and writing generally in use in the school system.
> (Miller, 2015, p. 33)

In truth there is endless debate about teaching reading and no consensus opinion about how to teach mainstream children, so it is likely to be far more difficult to arrive at a successful pedagogy for teaching children with IPDs.

Labels

The problem with any definition is one of identification, because without a firmly agreed definition there can be no proof of identity. This is not just an academic conundrum but determines who will receive the label and who will not. Despite a general reluctance from teachers, educationalists and clinicians to label individuals, and for them to be identified by that label, access to public money, support and even greater understanding and tolerance from teachers, employers and families is unlikely without the marker of a label.

> The question of definitions is not merely an academic issue, as definitions determine who receives the label that may act as a passport to accessing public money, appropriate support and possibly a more sympathetic

response from teachers, employers, supervisors and others. There is a tension between researchers' desires to classify difficulties clearly according to underlying causes and the political, social and economic implications of such categorisations.

(Morgan and Klein, 2000, p. 29)

However, labels are probably only the beginning of the process:

Acquiring support should not be the goal of the label but rather a signpost
(Reid and Kirk, 2001, p. 6)

Reid and Kirk (2001) also say that although a label is important it can also provide significant drawbacks with the potential to stigmatise those seeking employment. This fear can be seen in the interview conducted below with Erika.

Interview

Erika is currently at university in the final year of her BA degree. She was identified with dyslexia after a male friend, who was already identified, saw resonance of himself in her. She approached the university and was given an assessment (at no financial cost to Erika), and she now has a package of support in place (a learning contract), to help her with her final year of studies; this includes a laptop computer with voice recognition, spell checker, consideration in her written work and extra time in exams.

Primary school: Erika always had problems with spelling and reading and although she was given extra support with English by a teaching assistant it was never suggested that this could be dyslexia. Her parents were unaware of what to look for and so did not question the support offered by the school.

High school: Erika was always a hard worker but despite this never achieved the top sets in her subjects. However, she did manage to achieve C grades in all her GCSEs. She is the first in her family to go to university, but, in her own words, *did not think that I was clever enough to go to university*.

University:

I worked so hard in my second year but always got poorer grades than my friends even when we did group work, so we all had the same information but in written assignments they got better grades. However, I always did well in spoken presentations.

It was very frustrating, and I now feel resentful that because it was not picked up it could have been the difference between a few marks and it could have been the difference between getting into university or not.

I could easily have given up and often thought ... what is the matter with me?

It is such a sense of relief knowing now that it is not just me not being very clever. Things just do not go in. Sometimes I read but it does not go in. Recently I went to a museum with my boyfriend and was trying to read the information signs, but they did not make sense and I had to keep re-reading them. When friends show me things on their phone it takes me ages to read and understand what I am reading.

When I was a child it took me ages to learn to tell the time and everyone could tie their shoe laces before me.

I am quite athletic with running and things but find it hard to co-ordinate and hit a ball, although I did play hockey at school. I like to do practical things like cooking and baking.

I am not sure how I became so confident but my mum was always at home with us and encouraged me to read, she always read to me and with me.

Employment: Erika has recently completed a year on placement as part of her degree, interestingly she did not tell her employer about her difficulties. She was unable to explain that but did not want the employer to 'think less' of her.

> I might have told them if the employer had been a woman, but I did not think that he would understand.

When asked about future employment she did not think that she would want to tell employers in case she did not get the job, or they thought that she would be unable to cope with all aspects of the employment.

It is evident in the interview with Erika that in one sense a label can be really useful, directing limited resources and offering explanation for something that those with dyslexia frequently long for, as we see from the interview with John who has learned to believe in himself again.

Interview

John is sixty-four and a retired factory worker, having sprayed cars for a famous car manufacturer for thirty-five years. He and his wife had three children, all female and none had any problems at school. He now has five grandchildren, including Liam who is now nine years old and has recently been identified with dyslexia.

> I always struggled at school, in them days you got the stick when you could not do somethink and I got the stick every day. School days was a nightmare and I often bunked off and got into trouble. One day the policeman took me home for drawing on the walls of the nearby sweet shop. Me mam went mad and beat me to a inch of me life for bringing shame on her house by letting the neighbours see a policeman knocking on the door!
>
> The trouble was that I could not read very well and everything that we did in school seemed to need me to be able to read. All me mates could read and they could not understand what me problem was, eventually they started to bully me and making fun.

> Teachers told me ... and the rest of the class ... that I was thick and I frequently got brought to the front of the class as an example to all the other children of what happens to children who are 'thick' or don't work hard enough. I hated school and didn't really learn anything. It got even worse when I went to High School, I just did not seem to be able to understand the words on the page, even if I read them I could not understand what they said. I spent my whole life thinking that I was just stupid and that I would not amount to much.

Liam (John's nine-year-old grandson), struggles to read and to sequence; he still cannot tell the time and no matter how hard he tries he cannot remember his times tables. Liam is hopelessly disorganised and often does not arrive in school with the right equipment for the day or forgets his pens, books and clothing, which are left around the school for teachers and his parents to find. Fortunately for him a teacher spotted his problems and recommended that he was assessed for dyslexia which produced a positive result. Liam now has additional help with his work, tolerances from the staff and one-to-one reading sessions with the teaching assistant.

> I watched Liam struggling in school and I felt that I just knew what he was experiencing, it was terrible to watch as I did not know how to help. When he was tested and was told that he was dyslexic, it was like a big cloud lifting off me and I could see ... I do not know why I couldn't see it before ... that this was just the same as me. To be able to say that maybe I was not thick, stupid and useless, but that I was dyslexic was amazing ... there was a name for this thing that has followed me through life and it was not my fault.
>
> I recently paid to have a test meself and they said that I was dyslexic. It cost me over £300 for the test but it would have been worth twice that ... three times that ... and more ... to have known before. Even at my age it has made a big difference to know and understand ... me wife said that it did not matter ... but it did, it really did.
>
> Now Liam and I are learning to read together, he helps me and I help him ... we know that what we have is somethink that loads of others have and that we can manage it ... he can manage it through life.

An unnatural act

The ability to read in the UK is so prevalent that it is easy to forget that the majority of the world's population is functionally illiterate. Taking the reading process for granted is a grave mistake and begins with the misleading premise that everyone with appropriate intellectual capacity can be taught to read. That implies that if you cannot read you must be one of the following:

- Lacking in neurological, intellectual or perceptual capability
- Have never had the opportunity to be taught to learn to read
- Have had major psychological trauma, with social and emotional difficulties.

It is vital to remember that we are not 'born to read' and reading even in a very rudimentary format has only been a requirement for our brains for around four thousand years, which in evolutionary terms is miniscule. Gough and Hillinger (1980) even go so far as to title their article, in the *Bulletin of the Orton Society*, 'Learning to read: an unnatural act'. It is highly unlikely that our brains are inherently dyslexic, but it is highly probable that there are huge variations and differences between individuals in their cerebral functioning in the same way as there are variations and differences in our physical characteristics. These differences of brain function must deal with a reading process which is artificial and 'unnatural', and it is likely that they deal with these in slightly differing ways.

Cerebrodiversity is a term coined by Sherman and Cowen (2003) meaning that our brains are not all the same, with these differences it is likely that we learn differently and therefore potentially need to be taught differently. Sherman and Cowen (2003) suggest that there are rapid advances in neuroscience which show cellular differences in the brains of identified dyslexic individuals at a connectional and anatomical level.

REFLECT ON THIS

In evolutionary and historical terms dyslexia did not exist, not because it was not there, but because it was not a difficulty until there was a societal expectation for everyone to be literate. Difficulties in literacy are very real problems but the societal and emotional consequences are not, they result from the expectations of society and a lack of tolerance by others to those who are different.

1   Does having a label effectively say this person is not 'normal'?
2   People react to labels in different ways (both positive and negative); consider whether the addition of a label always leads to stereotyping and prejudicial attitudes to the individual concerned.

Prevalence

It must seem strange to many people that a condition which is so commonly discussed and so extensively researched cannot be accurately counted in the population as a whole. Earlier in this chapter it was highlighted that a definition was far from agreed and remains elusive and controversial, and as a consequence researchers in the field often base their research on different definitions, either operational or conceptual definitions, leading often to differing research findings and inevitably to further confusion. A conceptual, or constructive, definition is abstract and theoretical; it attempts to identify what the concept of dyslexia is and what it means. An operational definition, however, links that concept to the 'real' world, to enable it to be measured. An operational definition is therefore essential for reliable research to eliminate ambiguity. Contradictory criteria for a definition make it very difficult to compare samples in different research projects. This can be compounded still further when different languages and different orthographies are thrown into the mix. An operational definition once agreed could transform the conceptual definition into observable data. For this reason, no agreed figures or percentages of dyslexia prevalence can be reliably established. Whatever the exact prevalence of this condition (however it is defined), it is clear that there are a substantial number of individuals in this country and around the world who are both directly and indirectly affected. On a global stage generally, countries with a more transparent language (that is where each grapheme in the language corresponds consistently to one phoneme) exhibit less incidents of dyslexia than countries with languages which are opaque, when the correspondence between sound and letter is often unclear, such as English. Makita (1968) reported less than 1% of the population in Japan was dyslexic.

> One cannot expect to find an exact answer to this question [prevalence] as long as the concept of 'dyslexia' remains somewhat unclarified and controversial.
>
> (Klasen, 1972, p. 15)

In 1960 Silver and Hagin estimated that between 2–25% of the population of western cultures could be labelled dyslexic. A decade on and this was also the finding of Klasen (1972), but she also attempted to subdivide these statistics into severely affected and mildly affected cases. By 1981, Critchley set the average figure of 10% in British schools and by 2004 Miles and Miles estimated 3–6%. The British Dyslexia Association currently estimates approximately 10% with 4% severely affected in this country. However, Rice and Brooks (2004) say that without a reliable and agreed definition all these figures are probably at best a guess and are undoubtedly 'theoretically and technically contentious' (p. 20). This must be particularly so if the only criteria used for assessment is literacy based.

Another difficulty for those trying to assess the overall prevalence of dyslexia is that it is usually depicted on a sliding scale between mild and severe, so distinguishing any clear-cut moment at which dyslexia is present or not is very difficult. As Miles and Miles (2004) suggest 'nature is untidy' (p. 145) and clear cut-off points do not usually exist which probably explains why teachers often talk of a child's 'dyslexic tendencies' and 'grey areas'. It is not clear how these can be defined, especially when in some cases reading appears to be largely unaffected or what Miles and Miles (2004) call the 'compensated dyslexic' (p. 146).

They'll grow out of it!

Despite the lack of a conclusive definition we do know that this statement is just not true for someone with an IPD. They do not grow out of it, it is who they are and as much a part of them as the colour of their eyes or the shape of their ears. The IPD that they had as a tiny baby will probably influence their life experiences, expectations, friends and relationships and it stays with them, defining their life pathway through school, adolescence and into adulthood. All schools and colleges in the UK depend on the literacy of their students, and every subject taught makes a presumption that they are teaching literate individuals. These same schools and colleges rely upon exam and academic success for their future funding, so when an individual has difficulty with literacy they are at risk of failing all the academic subjects that society currently sees as important; imagine a situation where someone consistently experiences academic failure, imagine how they must feel. Even the more practical based options such as art, design and technology, food technology, engineering and sport have been 'academicised' and require the learner to pass written exams to be seen as successful. Often nothing that the individual with an IPD does in school or college is seen as achieving. The child and adolescent with an IPD probably starts to question whether they will continue to fail in life, in the same way that they have in education. What they may not know is that during that time many will have developed coping strategies to enable them to deal with life; they have probably developed resilience and the ability to 'take the knocks' and to get up and try again. These are valuable skills, essential for them if they are to become contributing members of society.

Despite there being a wide variation of operational definitions purported by the academics and 'experts' in the field there are also some interesting commonalities within these definitions. These make it easier to identify the condition, but not all are related to reading and literacy and many of the identifying criteria can be seen as advantages rather than difficulties. Probably the most common identifier is that it is familial, in other words there are often other close family members who have already been identified. Other common characteristics can be seen in the list below; however it is important to understand that this is not a tick sheet and I am sure that many of the things below are common to many people that you know, whether they have an IPD or not.

- The development of speech and pronunciation is often delayed and baby talk often persists beyond the time that would be expected.
- There is often a very literal interpretation of language: *Wait a minute* – they are expecting this to be exactly one minute!
- They often find it difficult to hear rhyme and alliteration, making it hard to clap or tap in time with a rhythm: King / Ring / Sing etc.
- There is often a general segmentation weaknesses and inability to blend sounds to make words: C-A-T cat or D-O-G dog.
- They often find the rules of language and grammar difficult (syntax): *I to the shops went* instead of *I went to the shops*.
- Occasionally there may be unusual word choices and substitution of words inappropriately: *tree house for tree trunk*, etc.
- Sound-letter correspondence is often difficult: *graphemes to phonemes*.
- Visual stress and light sensitivity can result in headaches, sore eyes and even nausea and dizziness.

- They may complain that the letters appear to move on the page or appear blurred, making it difficult to fixate on a word and eye strain results.
- Understandably they often deliberately avoid literacy-based activities.
- Having to concentrate so hard on the words can be tiring, resulting in a limited attention span.
- Short-term memory difficulties and sequential problems are very common, so a list of instructions is often forgotten or misinterpreted, and they can struggle to remember the names of things, particularly under any time pressure. Telling the time and remembering the days of the week, months of the year and past, present and future are often difficult.
- Finds colour concepts hard to establish.
- Often, they have personal organisation difficulties: never where s/he is supposed to be at an allocated time, always losing their possessions, etc.
- Unable to easily recognise shapes traced on to the skin with a finger.
- Cannot reliably recognise letters in their own name.
- Becomes confused when attempting to identify right and left.
- Difficulties with activities that involve spatial awareness such as jigsaws, nesting boxes, etc.
- Difficulties with gross motor control such as leg balance, walking backwards, etc.
- Often walks without crawling first (the bottom shuffler or tummy wriggler).
- Generally, has poor coordination.
- Difficulties with specific coordination such as catching a ball, kicking, throwing, hopping, skipping, etc.
- Finds it difficult to dress and undress, and often cannot remember the sequence of clothing. This is the child who puts their vest over their shirt or consistently puts shoes on the wrong feet, etc.
- Difficulties with fine motor skills such as grasping a pencil, using scissors, copying a pattern, drawing, manipulating buttons and tying shoe laces, etc.
- Often appears to be 'not trying' or 'not trying hard enough': the 'dreamer' who does not *appear* to be listening.
- The individual often has a poor self-image and lacks confidence in their abilities, experiencing good and bad days for no apparent reason.

Premature and early term babies with low birth weight (especially if they have been exposed to drugs and alcohol in utero), also appear to be more prone to IPDs. However there do appear to be some characteristics which could potentially be used to the advantage of the individual and society:

- Able to see the bigger picture: the holistic thinker.
- They often have excellent global visual processing skills, being able to recognise and memorise complex patterns.
- Able to make connections between patterns and images.
- Good spatial reasoning and able to manipulate a 3D image in their mind.

- Thinks in pictures rather than words.
- Increased peripheral vision: this could also be seen as a difficulty as it may make it harder to fixate and to suppress information from the periphery.
- They are often highly creative thinkers, curious about the world around them and beyond, making them great at problem solving, insightful and lateral thinkers.
- Many appear to have the ability to hear widely distributed sounds.
- Good long-term memory.
- Often verbally very articulate so potentially good communicators.

This list is certainly not exhaustive but is an amalgam of the most up-to-date thinking, no one person will have all of these, but where there are distinct clusters this may be an indicator for further expert assessment. There will also be huge variations in the severity of these indicators between individuals.

Chapter reflections

This opening chapter of the book demonstrates the confusion and controversy surrounding dyslexia from something as fundamental as the definition, to the advisability of labelling and prevalence; this confusion applies both to the professionals and the lay people alike. Clearly this makes the whole process of diagnostic assessment, dynamic teaching, intervention and resource allocation very difficult. Reid (2016) believes that this has led to each local education authority accepting differing approaches, which in turn has led to delays of assessment, conflicting advice for parents and variations in the levels of parental involvement and engagement.

Unfortunately, these differences of viewpoint also extend to the professionals working in the field; they probably all have competing pressures upon them which need to be prioritised according to their different perspectives. These may be financial pressures, commercial pressures, ideological, peer pressures, psychological, educational, party political and many more. These imperatives can at times bring the interested parties into conflict, causing yet more division and confusion.

Chapter two will examine the personal cost and some of the difficulties that many with IPDs and dyslexia undoubtedly have to cope with on a day-to-day basis, and what it really feels like to be dyslexic.

Further reading

Reid, G (2016) *Dyslexia: A Practitioner's Guide* (5th edn). Chichester: John Wiley and Sons.

This is now the fifth edition of this seminal text by Gavin Reid; it contains a vast amount of up-to-date material and thinking about dyslexia. Whether you are new to this area of research or an old hand, there will be something here for you. It is written in a language open to all who are interested in dyslexia, but also uses in-depth discussion to propose ideas, encourage debate and offer grounds for reflection. Reid readily combines theory with practice and his vast experience in the field ensures that this text is taken very seriously by all who read it. This is an essential text for anyone researching or writing about anything to do with dyslexia.

References

British Dyslexia Association (BDA) (2017) About the British Dyslexia Association. www.bdadyslexia.org.uk/about (accessed 11. 11. 18).

British Psychological Society (BPS) (1999) *Dyslexia, Literacy and Psychological Assessment: Report of a Working Party of the Division of Educational and Child Psychology*. Leicester: BPS.

Critchley, M. (1981). Dyslexia: an overview. In Pavlidis, GTh. and Miles, TR (eds), *Dyslexia Research and its Applications to Education*. London: J. Wiley & Sons.

Cutting LE, Clements-Stephens A, Pugh KR, Burns S, Cao A, Pekar JJ, Davis N and Rimrodt SL (2013) Not all reading disabilities are dyslexia: distinct neurobiology of specific comprehension deficits. *Brain Connect* 3(2):199–211. https://www.ncbi.nlm.nih.gov/pmc/articles/PMC3634135/ (accessed 30. 10. 18).

Dickins, C (1998) *Our Mutual Friend*. (Original publication 1869.) London: Heron Books.

Elliott, J and Grigorenko, EL (2014) *The Dyslexia Debate*. New York: Cambridge University Press.

Frith, U (1997) Brain, mind and behaviour in dyslexia. In Hulme, C and Snowling, M (eds) *Dyslexia: Biology, Cognition and Intervention*. London: Whurr.

Gough, PB and Hillinger, ML (1980) Learning to read: an unnatural act. *Bulletin of the Orton Society* 30: 179–196.

Hayes, C (2018) *Developmental Dyslexia from Birth to Eight: A Practitioner's Guide*. Abingdon: Routledge.

Higher Education Statistics Agency (HESA) (2017) Data and analysis. www.hesa.ack.uk (accessed 15. 11. 18).

International Dyslexia Association (2002) Definition of dyslexia. www.dyslexiaida.org/definition-of-dyslexia (accessed 11. 11. 20).

Klasen, E (1972) *The Syndrome of Specific Dyslexia*. Lancaster: Medical and Technical Publishing Co Ltd.

Luft, J. and Ingham, H. (1955), *The Johari Window: A Graphic Model for Interpersonal Relations*. Los Angeles: University of California Western Training Lab.

Makita, K (1968) The rarity of reading disability in Japanese children. *American Journal of Orthopsychiatry* 38: 599–614.

Miller, JF (2015) *Do You Read Me? Learning Difficulties, Dyslexia and the Denial of Meaning*. London: Karnac Books Ltd.

Miles, TR (2001) Reflections and research. In Hunter-Carsch, M (ed) *Dyslexia: A psychosocial perspective*. London: Whurr.

Miles TR and Miles E (2004) *Dyslexia and Mathematics* (2nd edn). Abingdon: Routledge.

Morgan, P (1896) A case of congenital word blindness. *British Medical Journal* 2: 1378.

Morgan E and Klein, C (2000) *The Dyslexic Adult: In a Non-dyslexic World*. London: Whurr Publications.

Nicolson, RI and Fawcett, AJ (1990) Automaticity: a new framework for dyslexia research? *Cognition* 35: 159–182.

Nosek, K (1997) *Dyslexia in Adults: Taking Charge of Your Life*. Maryland USA: Taylor Trade Publishing.

Reid, G (2016) *Dyslexia: A Practitioner's Handbook* (5th edn). Chichester: John Wiley and Sons.

Reid G and Kirk J (2001) *Dyslexia in Adults: Education and Employment*. Chichester: John Wiley and Sons Ltd.

Rice M and Brooks, G (2004) *Developmental Dyslexia in Adults: A Research Review*. London: National Research and Development Centre.

Rose, J (2009) *Identifying and Teaching Children and Young People with Dyslexia and Literacy Difficulties*. Nottingham: DCSF Publications.

Sherman, GF and Cowen, CD (2003) Neuroanatomy of dyslexia through the lens of cerebrodiversity: the value of different thinkers in our mists. *Perspectives* 29(2): 9–13.

Silver, AA and Hagin R (1960) Specific reading disability: delineation of the syndrome and relationship to cerebral dominance. *Comparative Psychology* 1(2): 126–134.

Tonnessen, FE (1997) How can we best define 'dyslexia'? *Dyslexia* 3: 78–92.

Xia Z, Hoeft F, Zhang L and Shu H. (2016) Neuroanatomical anomalies of dyslexia: disambiguating the effects of disorder, performance, and maturation. *Neuropsychological* 81: 68–78. www.ncbi.nlm.nih.gov/pubmed/26679527 (accessed 30.10.18).

2 Help! I'm drowning!

> You don't drown by falling in the water, you drown by staying there.
> Edwin Louis Cole (1922–2002)

Introduction

The quotation above is purported to be by Edwin Louis Cole (1922–2002), in one of his numerous sermons at the Christian Men's Network, but I believe that this quotation sums up how the person with dyslexia must feel when they are unsupported, unnoticed and afraid. This typifies the idea that it is not the difficulties that are experienced that cause problems, but when we are unable to come up with appropriate solutions. If we are able to keep swimming and keep our head above water, we can overcome all these challenges – as challenges they are. Resilience is so important to those with an information processing difference (IPD) and an understanding that when things are hard and you feel down, you do not need to stay down.

For most people who do not have an IPD or are not living closely with someone who has, it must be difficult to understand what it is like to live with the condition day in day out, for the rest of your life. For the child with undiagnosed dyslexia it often brings feelings of bewilderment, anxiety, fear and even shame, as they realise that they cannot do what *everyone else in the world* appears to be able to do so easily. As they mature into adulthood that sense of confusion, fear and shame is often heighted by the perceived need for concealment, secrets and feelings of anger and disempowerment.

This chapter will examine the personal cost, and some of the difficulties, that many with IPDs undoubtedly have to cope with on a daily basis, examining the powerful emotions, both positive and negative, of what it feels like to be dyslexic. Understanding the need to build determination and resilience will feature in this chapter and an examination of why some manage to do this, and build their lives successfully, and some do not.

Living with dyslexia

Despite the extensive research which has been conducted in recent years into the causes and aetiology of dyslexia, and an increasing awareness of the positive aspects of the condition, few who live with it initially talk about the positives when asked what it feels like to be dyslexic.

Interview

Eluned is sixteen years old and attending a Further Education College in Wales. She has enrolled upon a public services course level 2, not having achieved the GCSE grades that she had hoped for at school. Eluned is a first language Welsh speaker and attended a Welsh medium school from the age of five years. All her teaching was conducted in Welsh and her GCSE exams were all written in Welsh. Eluned's ambition is to join the police force.

> Although I struggled to read in my primary school my dyslexia was not picked up until I went to secondary school, even then it was not until the year eleven teacher suggested that I might have a problem. Until then I was always in the bottom set and thought that I was just 'thick' and 'stupid'. I certainly felt a failure. It was suggested to my mum that I was tested by the optician on a colorimeter machine. The optician prescribed glasses with tinted blue lenses. I really felt that these made a difference and I was able to read better. My mum had to pay for these, I think that she found this hard. I do not wear my glasses now as I am too embarrassed in front of other people in college, and I do not want people to know that I am a failure. The glasses just seemed to set me apart as people always wanted to know why I was wearing them.
>
> When I was at school, I didn't like reading in front of people, I felt nervous and really frustrated that others were able to read well, and I had failed to learn what they were all able to do. When I was at school, they also found that I was not good with numbers, and I failed both maths and English at GCSE with D grades. At school they gave me extra help, one to one with a teaching assistant twice a week, and this was helpful.
>
> At college they have said that I can have more time in exams, but the maths GCSE is all taught in English and I am finding this very difficult. I have asked if I can do this in Welsh, but they have not been able to arrange this. Learning maths in a second language is very difficult as the names of the operations and shapes and things are all different.
>
> When I join the police, I do not think that I will tell them about my learning difficulty because it may influence their decision about accepting me.

Eluned is an only child and to her knowledge neither parents or grandparents have dyslexia. It is interesting that Eluned not only refers to the difficulties that she has experienced, but also that she anticipates that she will continue to experience throughout her life. She refers to being a failure more than once in her interview, and despite being optimistic that she can have a career in the police, she believes that her condition will continue to put her at a disadvantage, with her need to keep it secret.

IPDs are probably the most common, and certainly the best-known, neurological differences impacting children and adults across the world, cross cultures, ethnic origins, genders and languages, yet it is probably one of the least well understood. Stories in the press of 'cures' and miraculous training programmes (usually enormously expensive), that will transform the individual in just a few weeks, also do not help the understanding of the condition. If, as we now believe to be the case, this is an inherited and developmental condition, then those who have it will have it for life. The individual with dyslexia will wake every morning with it from birth to death. That is not to say that they start each morning thinking *Oh dear! I am dyslexic, I am different*, but it does mean that they are likely to be affected by it in some way, every day, devising strategies to enable them to conduct their lives successfully and in a fulfilling manner.

It is important that a person is not defined by their differences, what we would now perhaps call discrimination, but that society is tolerant of difference and individuality. In the interview with Eluned (above) it is interesting to note that her concerns were all focused upon the reactions of the society that she lives in towards her, her school, her family, college and her future employment. I do not suppose that there are many people with dyslexia who start a conversation with *Hello, I'm Malcolm and I am dyslexic* any more than someone would start a conversation with *Hello, I'm Jane and I am a wheelchair user*. The only difference is that with any IPD it is 'hidden', it is not overtly obvious. Of course, this can be an advantage or a disadvantage, particularly when looking for employment, there are firms of architects in America, for example, who actively recruit those with dyslexia, believing them to be more creative and innovative in their designs. Dyslexia certainly can bring advantages and can assisted some in their search for employment, as their creativity and less usual ways of thinking may in fact define who they are.

Identification

The issue of identification and labelling has already been considered in chapter one but in this chapter, it is important to return to the issue from the perspective of how the label can make the individual with dyslexia feel. Morgan and Klein (2000) suggest that the reason for the assessment and identification of dyslexia is frequently different between children and adults. In children the identification and labelling is really concerned with discovering why a child is not learning and what support can be put in place to improve that learning potential, but in adults it is more likely that the reason for labelling will have more to do with litigation or eligibility for grants and concessions. However, in adults there is also the added reason of a quest to understand the often painful experiences that they had as a child, and a chance to dismiss the labels of *thick, stupid* and *lazy,* which have often defined their own self-concept and self-esteem over many years. Morgan and Klein (2000) believe that:

> It is thus often the starting point of huge changes in self-perception, learning experiences, ambitions, motivation and even personal relations.
> (Morgan and Klein, 2000, p. 21)

Of course, such a label can also bring feelings of anger and outrage for the way in which the education system has, as they see it, failed them or allowed them to feel that they had failed. Some have even attempted to seek redress through the courts, not necessarily for the financial compensation, but more for recognition and apology.

Case studies

What follows below are details of a very small number of cases of litigation which have taken place over the last decade, related to compensation for apparently negligent authorities and dyslexia. In reality there are many, many more and also many awaiting presentation to court.

> One pupil in Lincolnshire was awarded £23,343 from Lincolnshire County Council because it was deemed that his school had not fulfilled their statutory duty to identify his dyslexia.
>
> There was the case of Pamela Phelps who was awarded £45,650 in damages after she sued Hillingdon Council when she left school early because of her dyslexia and had to pay for private tuition for her GCSEs.
>
> Marcus Jarvis, who had no formal education after the age of twelve, took Hampshire County Council to court over their failure to provide a suitably adapted education for his dyslexia. He lost his case; however, as a result of the litigation the Law Lords stated that councils can be sued for failing to provide proper education.
>
> Robin Johnson was awarded £50,000 compensation from Stockport Metropolitan Borough Council, when he claimed that he did not reach his full academic potential, because the school that he attended failed to identify his dyslexia.

As indicated above, this is just a tiny proportion of the numbers of cases that legal representatives see each year related to dyslexia and other IPDs. As with any argument there are always at least two sides of a case and maybe you feel that, considering the potential number of individuals with this condition, we cannot afford, as a society, to be offering such compensation. However, it could also be argued that the money should be invested in the education system to provide training for teachers and education staff, with proper support in place to ensure that no one feels that they have to go through the lengthy and often tortuous route of the court system.

Trying to explain to someone who is not neurodiverse what it feels like for the individual with dyslexia is always going to be difficult, as any research relating to social and emotional development, feelings and experiences is always going to be imprecise and usually unscientific and unquantifiable. There are so many variables, such as the complexity of social data, the inability to clearly define concepts and causal relationships, social dynamics and many more, making it almost impossible to generalise results to the overall population.

> Another difficulty in researching this area, is that dyslexia is a developmental disorder which changes in its manifestations over time. It may be that social and emotional experiences change or fluctuate considerably over time and that circumstances, cumulative experiences and maturation all affect the likely outcome at a given point in time.
> (Riddick, 1996, pp. 32–33)

Self-image/self-esteem/self-concept

Self-image refers to how we see ourselves, or how we perceive ourselves in comparison to our ideal image of our self and in relation to how we believe others see us, so refers to what sort of person we believe that we are, and how we think others see us. Self-esteem, however, is usually defined as how we *feel* about ourselves, it is a global view of ourselves. At some point we all ask ourselves *who am I?* and it is these evaluations that coalesce into that global self-evaluation. Self-concept is usually described as a combination of these two with your ideal self, it is also usually domain specific, so how you feel about yourself as an academic, as an athlete, as a friend, as an attractive person, etc. According to Rogers (1961) we each have an image of ourselves as we are, and an image of our ideal self (Figure 2.1). When these come close together, we are likely to have a high self-esteem. However, those with low self-esteem can see a discrepancy between what they believe themselves to be and what they would like to be or think that they ought to be.

Rogers (1961) believes that the development of self-esteem is dependent upon two factors:

1. Unconditional positive regard: that is love and affection from others, especially those close to us.
2. Self-actualisation: that is fulfilling our potential and knowing that we can achieve to that potential.

When these two features are not present Rogers (1961) suggests that we are more likely to be vulnerable to low self-esteem (Figure 2.2). For most people low self-esteem results in a temporary emotional discomfort, but for some it can result in much more serious conditions such as mental health disorders and even clinical depression, implying that self-esteem is critical for both our physical and mental well-being.

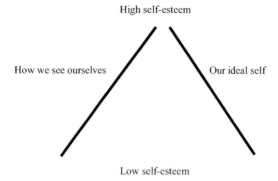

Figure 2.1 Self-esteem and the ideal self

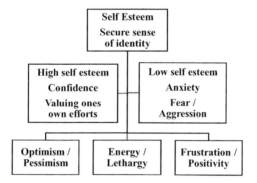

Figure 2.2 The hierarchy of self-esteem

Research by Burns (1982) showed that there was probably a strong connection between an individual's self-concept and their levels of educational achievement. However, Riddick (1996) reminds us that not all individuals with dyslexia have noticeable social and emotional difficulties, and the impact of an IPD on achievement and self-concept are broad ranging and highly variable. Some people are able to reach high levels of academic, physical and professional achievement, in spite of or even perhaps because of their dyslexia. Often the very difference in their thinking serves as a motivational force. At the other extreme some individuals feel defeated and make little effort to improve their situation. It is possible that these differences come down to how the individual sees their self or their self-image.

People generally gain in confidence every time they realise that they can achieve a particular outcome, so those with a strong self-image will see their goals as challenges to be achieved in the future. Conversely, each time they experience failure to achieve their goals, they risk feeling inferior and diminished in the eyes of their peers and are less likely to seek out further challenges and achievements. The individual with a low self-image will see these as hurdles, too high to climb, thereby stopping them from trying new things, afraid of trying hard for fear of failure. This constant experience of failure often leads to frustration, dissatisfaction, anger and even aggression.

There are so many influences upon the development of our self-image that the potential for its development to go 'wrong' is high. Reviewing the research into this area shows that some of the following may be influential, but there are clearly many more:

- Personality traits: shy, introvert, extrovert, strong willed, curious, sensitive, ambitious, anxious, etc. (many of which could arguably be genetic).
- Parental/carer expectations: is it important to your parents/carers that you are an achiever and can live up to their expectations?
- Life roles: are you a mother, a daughter, father, uncle, sister, etc. (how does society expect you to fulfil those roles)?
- Professional roles: are you a student, manager, teacher, factory worker, window cleaner, etc. (how does society expect you to fulfil those roles)?
- Leisure roles: are you a member of a committee or have community involvement?
- Age: self-image can be developmental and alter over time, according to maturation and life experiences.
- Gender: how you are expected to behave according to your gender and outward appearance of gender.
- Physical characteristics: a person of diminutive stature is unlikely to succeed in the basketball team, or someone with physical impairments or particular needs.
- Religion: there may be expectations upon the individual of life styles, behaviour and dress.
- Culture: someone brought up within a culture of success may react very differently to what they perceive as failure.
- Ethnic origin: feeling comfortable in your skin and with your own origins.
- Health: poor health can seriously inhibit the life experiences, expectations and ability to achieve.
- Abuse and neglect: this may interrupt the usual process of emotional and social development.
- Language: a non-English-speaking child in an all English-speaking school may struggle to achieve without support.
- Economic circumstances: poor economic circumstances can greatly inhibit life experiences and opportunities to achieve in a variety of skills.

These are only a few of the many potential influences upon the development of self-image and will probably impact upon each individual differently and uniquely. For example, when we have 'bad feelings' of fear, humiliation and frustration, often we deal with this by withdrawal from the situation, perhaps not wanting to communicate with anyone or we pass on our frustrations by being irritable and even aggressive, unfortunately often with the very people who are attempting to support us, and do not deserve this. For children this is often a carer or nearest 'safe' person. This is often referred to as emotional helplessness or learned helplessness.

Learned helplessness

The concept of learned helplessness was first developed by Seligman and Maier (1967) with their observational experiments on animals. A child who struggles to learn something such as literacy can begin to feel that nothing s/he does can have any impact on their ability to achieve. Learned helplessness is the point at which they stop trying to help themselves, because they feel that their existence is so out of their control that no matter what they do it will make no difference. Often this person feels that they are a victim of their own condition, and this can lead to serious feelings of anger and frustration or reach a point at which they just give up even trying. This is a phenomenon which occurs when we feel that we are in a negative situation and can see no escape from it; eventually even when the opportunity to escape does exist, the individual remains helpless.

Interview

Cathryn is sixteen years of age and attending a level two public services course at a further education college in Wales. She hopes to join the army as a dog handler, when she achieves level three. Cathryn is the youngest of six siblings, one older brother is dyslexic, and another has been identified as autistic. Although her father is not identified as dyslexic and fervently denies it, Cathryn believes that he too is dyslexic. Interestingly he refuses to even discuss this possibility.

> I was diagnosed in year six by the teacher and used the Toe by Toe programme with the teaching assistant. When I got to secondary school, I also got help from a teaching assistant.
>
> I know that I was 'thick' and tried to teach myself to read, but it was so hard. I noticed that when we were asked to write a story, everyone else was stuck, trying to think of things to write. I had lots to write about but had such difficulty with spelling it made it so hard and I couldn't get my thoughts on to paper so I was also stuck, but for different reasons. I love stories and can always think of new ideas and new plots.
>
> In primary school they made those with learning problems to do our SATS in a separate room; there were autistic children there that needed more help than I did. I didn't like it as it made me feel different. When I did exams in secondary school we were also in another room until GCSEs, when we were in the main hall, this was scary as I had never done that before. They made all those with difficulties sit in the two front rows … that was really embarrassing.

> I don't want the extra time and help as it is embarrassing and makes me feel 'not normal'. In secondary school I was bullied because I was 'not normal'.
>
> I wanted to be a vet but I am not bright enough, so I decided to be a dog handler in the army; two of my brothers and my dad were in the army. I don't think that the army would care about my dyslexia and it would not stop me getting in, but in other jobs it might be a problem. I like books, but I don't think that I have ever read a whole one. I find it so hard to concentrate, I get so distracted

Classical research into the area of self-esteem and self-concept comes from America with Harter (1987). She showed that the origins of difference in self-esteem come largely from parental and peer influences, which help to shape the value that an individual places on particular skills or qualities. The degree of importance that parents and peers place on a task, such as reading, sport, music etc., shapes the individual's internal expectations in that area. This is then further enhanced by the individual's experience of success or failure in that area. A child who is constantly told that they are a poor reader, stupid, thick and will not amount to much, is likely to have lower self-esteem than those who received praise and affirmation for their efforts. Harter (1987) found that it was particularly bad when a child perceives that parents' or carers' support is contingent upon being able to read well, play sport, achieve academically etc. Such experiences will clearly have an impact on a child's behaviour, so the child who is struggling with their IPD is likely to avoid the activities that tend to highlight these difficulties, refusing to try and avoiding books and activities that require this skill. They may even belittle the importance of reading and other children who read well. This child will often refuse to participate in reading activities, so that they are then seen as difficult by the teachers, *naughty* and *rebellious* and require chastisement or receive other negative consequences for their actions. The child who believes that s/he cannot read will behave very differently in school from the one who believes that they are good at reading, on the basis that if they do not attempt to read and actively avoid situations where reading is required, they will not fail. Alternatively, some children may try harder to read and thereby increase their anxiety levels about failure, which often extends to other areas of their life.

Learning to read and write is so important to our society, so the inability to do so is likely to have a profound effect on an individual's developing sense of identity. However, the struggle to read and write is not the only difficulty that those with dyslexia will face, and often the difficulties they experience in social settings can result in a vicious cycle of a poor quality of relationships and lack of confidence. Such difficulties can lead to anxiety, stress, fear of failing and embarrassment. This in turn can lead to isolation, as the individual shuns the social spaces where friendships and relationships are made.

In 1997 Chapman and Tunmer showed that there was a clear relationship between early reading ability and later self-concept; they believed that success at school (however that is interpreted) is important to the development of positive self-concept, and high self-esteem could have an effect on later reading ability (Figure 2.3).

Those with high self-esteem expect to succeed, whereas those with low self-esteem expect to fail. Such individuals tend to blame themselves for their inability and when they do achieve success, they believe that it is clearly not to do with their own abilities or efforts, but down to environmental factors or just plain 'luck'. This fits into Seligman and Maier's (1967) concept of learned helplessness.

Social and emotional consequences

One of the difficulties when researching the social and emotional consequences of dyslexia is defining the terms social and emotional difficulties, and even the word dyslexia itself (as you have already seen in chapter one); these terms are very imprecise. The range of attributes, skills, personal characteristics and features of identity make defining and measuring social and emotional issues very difficult. They are often lying on a continuum, and frequently there is an overlap between antisocial behaviour and mental health disorders. Another problem with researching self-esteem and self-concept is that, as Riddick (2010) suggests, a child who has been well supported at home and school may cope better with the challenges of the condition than one with less support and understanding, and can develop higher levels of resilience to the occasions of failure. A further difficulty is that as a developmental condition it is likely to change over time with maturity and increased life experiences.

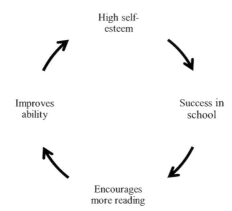

Figure 2.3 Cycle of success and high self-esteem

> It may be that social and emotional experiences change or fluctuate considerably over time and that circumstances, culminative experiences and maturation all affect the likely outcome at a given point in time.
>
> (Riddick, 2010, p. 35)

It is important not to assume that all individuals with an IPD will automatically have social and emotional problems as many do not. Riddick (2010) suggests that educational establishments such as schools and colleges pose the greatest threat to the development of high self-esteem and high self-concept, as it is difficult to escape or avoid the things that we are less good at, especially as literacy is essential for all things learned there. In schools and colleges, you are subjected to overt assessment and potentially negative feedback, which individuals respond to in different ways; some are able to ignore and discount, but others are more sensitive to harsh criticism and failure depending upon personality and levels of learned resilience. This in turn can further lower self-esteem, resulting in giving up more easily when undertaking a task of difficulty, they can become fearful of approaching such a task and will even avoid a situation where failure may potentially occur and they feel that they have low expectations of their chances of success. In other words, their level of resilience is low.

Resilience

According to the Oxford Dictionary to be resilient is to be *able to recoil, spring back into shape after bending, stretching or being compressed. Able to recover quickly from difficult conditions.* It is a term which is also frequently used to refer to how an individual is able to deal with any crisis in their lives. This implies that it is a reaction to a one-off, short-lived experience, whereas being born with any particular condition which sets you apart from the rest of the population is certainly not a crisis, it is not an acute condition but a chronic state. This implies that what would normally be an emotional process to help us to cope with the most traumatic times in our lives, for the individual with an IPD needs to be employed every day; this is unlikely to be helpful, or even possible. People with any long-term functioning differences need to be able to work with their difficulties and not just skirt around them, lurching from one crisis to another.

Listening to so many people with IPDs during the writing of this book, it is striking that what appears to be the single most important determinant of whether an individual thrives emotionally or not is resilience. The ability to come to terms with their condition is often determined by the presence of someone in their life who is supportive and encouraging, someone who believes in their abilities and is not obsessed with disabilities. Usually this would be a parent or carer, but in some instances could be a special teacher, or in the case of adults, an understanding partner. Such external factors certainly appear to support the development of resilience and the adoption of positive self-concept and optimistic thinking. Resilience in this context means the ability to learn to cope with adversity. A review of research by Haft et al. (2016), showed that children with strong family cohesion are likely to have a higher self-concept than those with weaker relationships. Strong relationships, such as peers or a best friend, supportive teachers and teacher mentorship, where teachers are caring and available, can help to create a belief that the individual has the capacity to adapt to adversity, it can foster a growth mindset (Dweck, 2007), that is a belief that you can develop and improve and achieve (Figure 2.4).

Interview

Aashirbaad is a first language English speaker of Asian heritage, now in his thirties. He recalls his traumatic time in British school at a time when he was not aware of his dyslexia. Sadly, this interview was typical of many that were conducted for this book.

> I found school very difficult because I didn't understand what was going on. I couldn't follow what was said, and the others in the class just called me 'thick' and 'stupid' and 'lazy'; when I look back I suppose that this was just bullying, but at the time it was not seen like that, and I suppose inside I just agreed with them, because after all, I couldn't do the work or follow the lessons. I didn't really have any friends, so I became a bit of a loner, preferring my own company and shutting myself away. I felt different to anyone else, and even though I was good at sport and quite creative, it didn't seem to matter. I became so pent-up and frustrated and sometimes even, I'm ashamed to say, aggressive. I remember one day when the

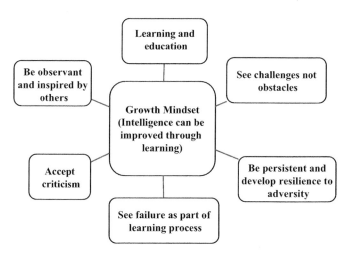

Figure 2.4 The growth mindset
Inspired by Dweck (2007)

teacher was shouting at me, his head was so close to me that I could feel his spit on my face, and as he turned to go I picked up a chair and threw it across the room where it broke on the floor. I got into so much trouble, so it was easier just to withdraw rather than to fight. The other children left me alone for a while after that, I think they were scared of me, of what I might do. I suppose I was just fighting back. When I was at home sometimes, I would try to read, but would end up screaming and tearing up the book or punching the wall.

Behaviour

Issues of low self-esteem and other social and emotional difficulties are in many children likely to lead to issues with behaviour, particularly for a child in a school environment which is so completely literacy focused (PACFOLD, 2007). A very influential study in this field conducted by Rutter et al. (1970) appeared to show that in the Isle of Wight approximately a quarter of children with reading difficulties also had issues with varying levels of antisocial behaviour. Further and more recent longitudinal studies such as those by Heiervang et al. (2001) have also shown a strong correlation between dyslexia, reading difficulties and antisocial behaviour. This study also appeared to show that levels of frustration and demoralisation build and increase over time, leading to unwanted social behaviour or withdrawal, disengagement and over compliance (the latter are more likely to be overlooked in a busy classroom environment). Riddick (2010) suggests that this leads to anxiety, loss of confidence and low motivation.

> [In school] they thought I was stupid and arrogant, they believed I could have done the work if I tried. The headmaster – S Kelton, a horrid man – used to cane me for not being able to spell. He made me stand up in class and he would embarrass me because he thought I was getting the words wrong on purpose, no one thought about dyslexia in those days. I thought I was stupid.
> (David Bailey CBE, world renowned photographer in Rooke, 2016, p. 27)

Interestingly, for some people the school and academic environment is a godsend, as is illustrated by Darcey Bussell CBE, the world-famous ballerina:

> I became more anxious about my dyslexia when I was 18 and out in the 'real world'. I felt as if I'd lost the protection of school and people would notice more. I hated the pressure of having to write a cheque in front of someone. I wondered how I could pretend I could do this and hide my problem with writing.
> (Darcey Bussell CBE in Rooke, 2016, p. 71)

REFLECT ON THIS

Just for a moment consider something in your own life that you are not very good at … maybe you cannot swim, perhaps you find it hard in a party situation, maybe you are a really bad cook, you are afraid of heights, etc.

1   How does it make you feel to know that you are not good at something?
2   Does it depend on the context at the time?
3   How do you think others see you when they know about your difficulties?
4   Do you try to avoid situations where this 'failing' may be exposed?
5   Do you manage to conceal your difficulty or do you 'brazen it out'?

Bullying

Much has been written about bullying, although there is no clearly defined legal definition of bullying, but government documents usually define it as behaviour which involves repeated intent to harm someone, either physically or emotionally, and a real or perceived power imbalance. This could be child on child, adult on adult, or more concerningly the adult on child, specifically teacher on child. This can take place in school or the workplace or today increasingly events take place online, in the form of cyber bullying, so can come directly into the home. It is generally recognised that certain groups are more susceptible than others, and those with a condition such as an IPD may find it difficult to correctly spell or write texts or become involved in social media, and others may pick up on this and tease them or send nasty text messages, spread rumours on social media, or even impersonate them and sign up for unwanted items or services that can get someone into trouble. Those who already have a low opinion of themselves may be more vulnerable to bullying and become victims, further lowering their self-esteem. Any child can experience bullying, but certain factors may make it more likely. Alexander-Passe (2010) suggests that there is evidence pointing to those with dyslexia being more susceptible to being bullied at school, he suggests that this in turn can lead the bullied becoming the bully, in order to increase their own self-esteem and feelings of status.

A recent interpretive phenomenological study by Shaw and Anderson (2018) considered the experiences of eight medical students/junior doctors, with dyslexia. They found that experiences of helplessness and hopelessness were common, with the fear of stigmatisation and feelings of inadequacy. Those involved talked of bullying, rejection and belittling from other medical students; some called them 'fake dyslexics', invoking feelings of victimisation and self-consciousness. Such bullying can be deeply wounding and discriminatory to someone with an already heightened sensitivity. Paradoxically some experienced a sense of achievement at overcoming the challenges; it made them work harder to overcome their difficulties, seeing it as a challenge with a need to prove that people were wrong about them, thereby using dyslexia to their advantage.

Whatever the circumstances, anyone who is being bullied faces enormous challenges every day; they feel that people are being judgemental, and this can provoke feelings of anger, isolation, worthlessness and loneliness which can affect both mental and physical health.

A non-dyslexic world

A non-dyslexic world is hard to describe when it really is just the accepted environment that we all live in. However, try to imagine how it must be on a day-to-day basis for the dyslexic person living in a world of literacy. A non-dyslexic world is clearly one which has an expectation that everyone over the age of five years of age is literate. Imagine for a moment living in a world where everyone expects you to be able to talk, or see, or hear ... you do not look any different from anyone else, so everyone that you meet expects that you can achieve certain things in a certain socially accepted way, and when you cannot it must be your fault ... stupid, lazy, pretending for effect, etc. There are so many barriers even to a fulfilling social life that those who are literate take for granted.

- There is a lack of information, so you arrive on the wrong day, the wrong time, etc.
- You find it hard to read letters, texts, e-mails so you are not sure where to go for that interview or even who to ask for.
- Even your school reports become a mystery – you know that they are talking about *you,* but you do not know what they say.
- There is a fear of rejection and ridicule, so you avoid going to places, meeting people and socialising.
- New technologies such as computers, smart phones, iPads and the like are difficult to use and understand.
- You cannot read and understand your rights and what benefits you might be entitled to, potentially leading to poverty and unemployment.
- Instructions on food packaging are difficult to follow and you find it hard to assess the cooking times.
- You cannot follow instructions so get lost, especially when distinguishing left from right.
- Jokes, puns and sarcasm are hard to understand, especially when they are written down, such as texts and online – *everyone laughs and I laugh because they are laughing, but I cannot understand what it says.*
- You do not seem to fit in with your peer group.

Chapter reflections

It would be entirely reasonable to expect that, due to the increased research interest and understanding of this condition, children would by now be having a more positive experience of their school days. Unfortunately, this does not always appear to be the case. Listening to children's experiences, albeit in a very anecdotal way, I still hear the anguish and often fear that they experience. Research by Burden (2005) suggested that children with dyslexia in a mainstream school recorded significantly lower on a scale known as Myself as a Learner (MALS) than children not identified as dyslexic. MALS is a research tool to assess how individuals perceive of themselves as learners and problem solvers, their academic self-concept. Burden's research also showed that when children with dyslexia were moved from a mainstream school to a specialist dyslexia unit their MALS score showed significant improvements.

> School was awful. For years I would have this horrible stomach ache, a dull pain inside me. Imagine a 16-year-old kid walking round with a six-year-old boy's anxieties in his stomach. I looked confident on the outside and was terrified on the inside. Words and letters confused me from the very beginning of primary school to the end of high school. I saw the other children progress while I was left drowning.
> (Kenny Logan, Scottish International rugby player and businessman in Rooke, 2016, p. 119)

Having this sort of IPD is a bit like a three-legged dog, he cannot run as fast as the other dogs, he cannot play as well with them, as he can never catch them up, but he learns ways and strategies around his condition, and can live a fulfilling and satisfying life, bringing joy and inspiration to those around them. He can still be a guide dog, the sniffer dog, the therapy dog, or just the well-loved and highly valued companion.

You have already read in chapter one of the large number of very successful members of society with dyslexia, who have succeeded despite of or perhaps because of their condition, so there is clearly something about some people with the dyslexic brain, that creates individuals with unparalleled creativity, design skills, spatial awareness and perception. It could be that they are more suited to the preliterate past, when exploration, pioneering and a spirit of adventure were more valued than literacy. Wolf (2008) questions whether in the future those with IPDs will re-emerge as the most valuable brain types, as three-dimensional and multi-dimensional symbols and technologies take over from books and technology steeped in reading.

Not all people with dyslexia have amazing talents, but they can all fulfil their potential with the right acknowledgement and intervention; this cannot be achieved by a one-size-fits-all, or by intimidating, humiliating and rejecting these individuals, just because society does not know how to respond to them. If these individuals learn differently then perhaps society needs to treat them differently and teach them differently.

In the next chapter you will read how families cope having someone with an IPD in their midst and the cost to them both financially and emotionally. The chapter will focus on the importance of encouragement, respect and unrelenting support, to developing the levels of resilience needed to improve the life chances of those with IPDs.

Further reading

Rooke, M (2016) *Creative Successful Dyslexic: 23 High Achievers Share Their Stories*. London: Jessica Kingsley Publications.

This book does exactly what it says, it showcases twenty-three people who have been successful in their field, despite or perhaps because of their dyslexia. It certainly demonstrates that dyslexia and IPDs do not necessarily have to hold back those with the determination and resilience to succeed. This book also demonstrates well that dyslexia is for life and will always have an impact (positive and negative), upon the individual. This book certainly contains some inspirational stories of people overcoming their difficulties and gives an important insight into how it really feels to be dyslexic and the inner strength and resilience needed to achieve their goals.

References

Alexander-Passe, N (2010) *Dyslexia and Mental Health*. London: Jessica Kingsley.
Burden, R (2005) *Dyslexia and Self-concept*. London: Whurr.
Burns, R (1982) *Self Concept Development and Education*, London: Holt, Rinehart and Winston.
Chapman, JW and Tunmer, WE (1997) A longitudinal study of beginning reading achievements and reading self-concept. *British Journal of Educational Psychology* 67: 279–291.
Cole, EL (1922–2002) Ed Cole Library. www.edcole.org/ (accessed 20. 12. 19).
Dweck, C (2007) *Mindset: The New Psychology of Success*. Stanford, USA: Ballantine Books.
Haft, SL, Mayers, CA and Hoeft, F (2016) Socio-emotional and cognitive resilience in children with reading disabilities. www.ncbi.nlm.nih.gov/pmc/articles/PMC5058360/ (accessed 20. 11. 19).
Harter, S (1987) The determinants and mediational role of global self-worth in children. In Eisenberg, N (ed.), *Contemporary Topics in Reply to Developmental Psychology*. New York: John Wiley.
Heiervang, E, Stevenson, J, Lund, A and Hugdahl, K (2001) Behavioural problems in children with dyslexia. *Nordic Journal of Psychiatry* 55(4): 251–256.
Morgan, E and Klein, C (2000) *The Dyslexic Adult: In a Non-dyslexic World*. London: Whurr Publications.
PACFOLD (Pacific Centre for Flexible, and Open Learning for Development) (2007) *Putting a Canadian Face on Learning Disability*. Learning Disabilities Association of Canada. www.pacfold.ca (accessed 22. 12. 19).
Riddick. B (1996) *Living with Dyslexia*. London: Routledge.
Riddick. B (2010) *Living with Dyslexia: The Social and Emotional Consequences of Specific Learning Difficulties* (2nd edn). Oxon: Routledge.
Rogers, C (1961) *On Becoming a Person: A Therapist's View of Psychotherapy*. Boston: Houghton-Mifflin.
Rooke, M (2016) *Creative Successful Dyslexic: 23 High Achievers Share Their Stories*. London: Jessica Kingsley Publications.
Rutter, M., Tizzard, J and Whitmore, K (eds) (1970) *Education, Health and Behaviour*. London: Longman and Green.

Seligman, M and Maier, S (1967) Failure to escape traumatic shock. *Journal of Experimental Psychology* 74: 1–9.

Shaw, SCK and Anderson, JL (2018) The experiences of medical students with dyslexia: an interpretive phenomenological study. *Dyslexia: An International Journal of Research and Practice* 24 (3).

Wolf, M (2008) *Proust and the Squid*. Cambridge: Icon Books.

3 The cost to family and friends

Introduction

'I hate you' is a phrase commonly heard in families with children. The ubiquitous tantrum when frustration and anger reach boiling point and explode into noisy arguments, flouncing out and even physical violence. Books on child development often warn parents of the 'terrible twos', but this is certainly not a phenomenon confined to the very youngest children. Teenage tantrums are often provoked by the frustrations felt in the young person towards themselves and others, with their feelings of powerlessness and inability. This is quite normal behaviour, but imagine experiencing these frustrations day in day out, as you feel unable to do what others appear to find so simple.

Living with someone with dyslexia can be difficult, the concept that dyslexia is just about reading is quite wrong, and living with someone whose level of organisation is so poor can be challenging, their homes, rooms, workspaces may be chaotic and untidy, which some people find hard to live with. They have to work harder than others to achieve a seemingly everyday task, so may be more tired than you might expect. It can be wearing to be constantly asked how to spell something, to proofread material, repeatedly asked for phone numbers and shopping lists, etc. Their poor time keeping may mean that they miss appointments, or don't turn up to meet you when they say they will. They may not be able to adapt when the usual daily routine is disrupted. It can be frustrating to live with someone whose short-term memory is so poor, when they forget to put out the bins on the right day, or cannot remember instructions given to them to go left instead of right at a junction.

This chapter will examine some of the costs and benefits to families and friends of an information processing difference (IPD). Parents and carers have a key role to play in helping their children come to terms with what nature has given them, developing resilience and coping with stress and anxiety; however, there will often be recriminations and feelings of guilt and blame within families, even feelings of inadequacy in their parenting skills, with parents having to juggle the demands of extra expenses and time commitments, with the needs of other family members, work and even recreation or 'down time'.

Perhaps the most important issue for parents and families is one of recognition and acceptance. That is not to say that their child or family member needs to be formally assessed or identified, but rather that there is a recognition that we are all different, acceptance of who we are is essential to our well-being and health. That acceptance and managing to look at the positive rather than the negative is probably the key to the generation of effective learning and achievement.

> When Edison invented the electric light, he failed 1,2000 times before he got it to work. When a journalist asked him 'How did you deal with 1,200 failures?' Edison replied 'I did not fail 1,200 times. I was successful at finding 1,200 ways the light bulb didn't work!'
>
> (Nosek, 1997, p. 30)

The middle-class disease

The 'middle-class disease' was a phrase commonly heard in the 1960s, 1970s and 1980s about dyslexia. The argument was that there were more children from middle-class homes (whatever that may mean) who were identified with this condition, than children whose parents were in a group with a lower socio-economic status. It was largely teachers, and other so-called experts, who believed that children who struggle with literacy were just stubborn, lazy or reticent to learn. Parents of children who came from literate and supportive homes were often concerned at the distress of their children, when they saw that they were experiencing some sort of barrier to learning that schools often did not acknowledge. The most articulate families would broach this with their child's teacher; they had the confidence and self-assurance to talk persuasively to headteachers and local education authorities, until they were heard and managed to achieve appropriate support and intervention for their child. These same parents were often in financially secure positions to be able to afford to have their children adequately assessed by an educational psychologist, often at huge personal financial cost. They were able to achieve an assessment and identification which could not be ignored by local education authorities and schools, forcing them to accept the dyslexia label and using legislation and the Special Needs Code of Practice, to ensure appropriate support for their child. Many felt that even then their child did not receive the appropriate structures in their education that they needed to succeed in the state system, and they withdrew them from school, either to the private sector or even start to home school their children. The distress that they saw in their child, and the downward spiral that they observed in their social and emotional development, their behaviour and academic learning, convinced them that this was the best path for them to follow. As a consequence, there was a steep rise in schools within the private sector offering specialist education for a range of IPDs, with smaller classes and teachers, who, parents believed, were better able to understand the needs of their children. This came at a huge financial cost and clearly was a route open only to those with sufficient disposable income to be able to afford this. The average cost of an independent educational psychologist assessment at today's rate is between £300–400. This, as can be seen in the following interview with Veronica, is multiplied still further when a family has more than one child with an IPD. In Veronica's case the children went on to university, so needed further adult assessments, which resulted in Veronica paying for six educational psychology assessments.

Interview

Veronica realised that she was dyslexic when her own children were identified; she has three children, now in their 20s and 30s, all have been identified as dyslexic.

1. Male (1) is now an investment analyst and works with numbers and maths, which he has never found to be a problem. He copes by developing strategies to enable him to read and write reports.

When he attended primary school, he was identified informally and Veronica was told that the costs involved in formal identification were too high for the school budgets, and they did not feel that they had the expertise to help. In desperation Veronica paid for a formal psychological assessment and when dyslexia was identified in her son she moved him to a local independent school, which specialised in supporting children and families with dyslexia, he subsequently went to university and achieved a first class honours degree.

2. Female, now a social worker, was assessed with mild dyslexia; she attended the same independent school as her brother and received support, she also went on to gain a first class honours degree at university.

3. Male (2), diagnosed with severe dyslexia, he also attended the independent specialist school, and went on to do a degree in agriculture. Veronica noticed that at the local further education college he had received a great deal of support to enable his learning, but when he went to university support was minimal, and comprised mostly of support in terms of a Dictaphone, laptop, etc. Son number two still requires support and is in constant touch with Veronica to ask about spellings and for her to read his reports. Often these are just basic words such as 'road' and 'car'. He is very talented at fixing things, particularly large farm vehicles. He is popular and highly articulate, caring and understanding; however his mother believes that dyslexia *definitely* limited his career and career choices. He needs considerable support to write a CV and tires easily. He finds it difficult to read the replies to his job applications, so has in the past missed opportunities for interviews, as he has not understood the response letter from the employer. Often it is Veronica who has to write his applications, as he lacks the confidence even to apply.

There can be tensions created between him and his older brother who is earning far more than son (2); he understands his brother's difficulties, so will offer to pay for him to go to events, but this can be resented.

As all three children needed an assessment in primary school and a further assessment before going to university Veronica has paid for six assessments in total costing the family almost £2,000, just to have the condition recognised. There was no financial help with this cost available.

As a child Veronica felt that she was more able than the teacher suggested. She was not engaged with school, and was often thrown out of class for being disruptive or the class clown; however, she loved to do activities with her hands and became the only girl in the school to take metalwork and technical drawing, she was top of the class particularly with Airfix models. Her maths was very poor and times tables and telling the time were particularly difficult, although she was always able to manage money. Even now she often arrives as much as an hour early for an appointment, for fear of not making it on time.

Veronica has a very supportive family, even though they did not understand that she was dyslexic, and when she left school at the age of sixteen, she started a job in technical drawing and became a graphic designer. Now she writes reports, reading and rereading them constantly to check that they make sense, she uses words that she is confident with, so because she muddles up simple words such as 'can' and 'can't', she will always write 'cannot' to be sure. She just avoids her problem words. Her early career was all based on doing things, and it was not until she was thirty years of age that she needed to write.

> Dyslexia definitely, definitely, definitely, limited my career and it was only with very hard work that I was able to achieve. I had three jobs, and with determination and resilience maintained a 'can do' attitude. There was a lack of expectation placed upon me, but I think I was made more resilient because of it.

Veronica has an identical twin who also has dyslexia, although she has never been formally identified. She runs her own business, but frequently has problems with letters and emails and needs her employees to sort them out for her.

The average cost per year of a child attending even a less prestigious fee paying school is, in today's climate, approximately £17,000 per year, that is likely to be at a cost of £119,000 just for secondary schooling alone, if the child remains in school to sixth form.

Looking at these enormous sums of money it is easy to see that a disproportionate number of children from wealthier homes were, and probably still are, identified as dyslexic, hence the label the 'middle-class disease'. Teachers and those who were ignorant of the implications of the condition genuinely believed that this was middle-class parents who were so ashamed of their child's struggle with reading, so overwhelmed with guilt, that it was somehow their fault, that they needed a label, a syndrome, a condition to excuse their perceived parenting inadequacies. These teachers believed that literacy could be achieved by anyone with an appropriate level of intelligence and refused to accept dyslexia. This of course meant that many children with less articulate, financially stable parents were left to struggle and labelled as stupid, lazy and unteachable.

The Times Educational Supplement in 1998 published an article by Ghouri, which claimed that:

> Mothers from low income families are too intimidated by schools and teachers to ask for their help with their children's learning.
> (Ghouri, 1998, p 4)

Ghouri claimed that these parents did not find their child's school a welcoming place and they were not parent friendly spaces.

Parent friendly

All schools are now expected to have a parent partnership policy in place to engage with parents, families, carers and the local community. The SEND Code of Practice (Department for Education and Department of Health, 2015) emphasises the importance of such partnerships to the child's learning and development, when the relationship is interactive and dialogic. Parents need to move from being passive receivers of educational services, to being active participants and advocates for their children's rights. In this way parents and schools can co-construct the support and educational provision that is right for their child. However, to be able to do this, parents have to have the time, and be prepared to put in considerable effort, with the cultural and social capital necessary.

It is so important that schools and teachers are aware of the cost to parents coming into school, to express their concern about their child's progress. This is particularly so for families with a child who is at risk of an IPD. The familial nature of these conditions means that it is highly likely that the parents have also experienced an unsuccessful period in school. Their relationship with schools and education is already very tainted. They may remember the disasters and humiliation they suffered in school, they may have spent their school days being verbally and even physically abused by teachers, and at the extreme, may have experienced suspension and expulsion from school or schools, which could have even resulted in school phobia. Some believed that their relationship with schools and education was over for good, but now find themselves having to confront their fears and go into a school environment to talk to teachers again. The courage and conviction that this requires is probably inestimable, and they may have spent many days, weeks and months putting off the moment when they had to step over the threshold of the school, and all the distress and anguish comes flooding back. By the time that such a parent finally reaches the teacher to speak, it is difficult to imagine that they can put into words their genuine fears and concerns about their own child. The bravery of such parents to open that dialogue with the school is immeasurable. Many such parents find this just too stressful and however much they want to support their children and prevent them experiencing the same distress and anguish that they suffered, the cost to their own lives is just too great. For these children, unless they are lucky enough to encounter another supportive and understanding adult, such as a teacher, teaching assistant or family member, their school experience is likely to be negative, and, in some cases, unbearable.

Some years ago, I worked with the Adult Literacy and Basic Skills Unit (ALBSU), running programmes for parents with low literacy skills; many were clearly undiagnosed dyslexics. My one abiding memory of this time was the shame and guilt that so many of these parents felt; they had spent their whole lives trying to conceal their difficulties. I could not believe the number who confided to me that even their own husbands, wives or partners did not know that they could not read. Imagine spending a lifetime concealing something as fundamental as this, from even those that you love and trust the most in this world. The stress and anxiety that this must engender, the lies and deception that this must generate, the guilt, fear and angst must be almost unimaginable.

Parents of children with an IPD often report that they face rejection from schools and teachers when they first express concern. Some of the following comments were heard during interviews:

> *No need to worry, she is just a little slower to grasp the reading.* [This is such a passive stance and according to Shaywitz (2005) typically assumes that all will work out in the end]
>
> *Don't try to compare him with the other children in the class this is divisive and unhelpful.* [Who else does a parent have to compare them with?]
>
> *He just needs to concentrate more!*
>
> *She is so disruptive in class it's no wonder she struggles to read.* [Does anyone bother to find out *why* they are so disruptive?]
>
> *He's got plenty of time to catch up.* [To the mother of an eight-year-old]
>
> *We don't compare children nowadays it's useless.* [To the mother of a third child, comparing him with her experiences of his siblings]

I am quite sure that the teachers that made these comments, made them in what they saw as in the best interests of the child. They no doubt wanted to appear friendly and non-intimidating, but the picture that the parents paint is very different. Parents often feel that it was rude and presumptuous to criticise or question the 'experts', as they see it. Parents also comment that there was a disparity between what the school said in their policy documents, and what they actually did. From these comments it is clear that some parents appear better able to exercise their rights to support, financial resources and legal representation than others. Being a parent is probably the hardest job that anyone can undertake, and it certainly does not come with a manual!

> Parents increasingly feel that they are in a position to choose the best care and education for their children, a good value for their money in a competitive market where schools and teachers are perceived as being 'service

providers'. In this context, some parents see themselves as the main decision-makers in terms of selecting the education services they deem appropriate for their children.

(Hartas, 2006, p. 78)

The untold secret

Foss (2016) talks about the struggle of a parent to admit their own dyslexia to their children. As a young child we frequently believe that our parents are all knowing and infallible, so for some to make the revelation to young children that they too struggled to read (and possibly still do) can be a very difficult admission.

> A good friend who is a national public advocate for specific learning disabilities recently called me in tears when he learned that his own child was dyslexic: he was terrified that the boy would be put through the same harassment he had endured and even more scared to admit to his son that he was dyslexic as well.
>
> (Foss, 2016, p. 19)

Foss (2016) is also dyslexic and claims that he spent thirty years attempting to hide his dyslexia. He believes that any feelings of shame surrounding dyslexia probably start with the relationship between parents and their child. Not wanting a child to have the same traumatic educational experience that they did can, in some circumstances, make parents reluctant to have a formal assessment and label for their child. They may even be concerned that this will formally identify their child as 'not quite perfect', or even worse 'not quite normal'. Once that label is applied there is a feeling that it can never be reversed, and this can carry a stigma. Foss (2016) talks about parents in the USA who ask the teachers not to talk about their child's dyslexia, or reveal it to other parents; this can in turn lead to denial with parents refusing to admit that their child may need support or additional guidance. This can also lead to an over-anxious and pressurising parent, as they are so aware of how hard it was for them, and do not want similar difficulties and misery to be heaped upon their own child. In turn this can lead to breakdowns in relationships, when they become so fraught and anxious that either parent or child loses patience and tempers flare.

The home learning environment

Babies emerge from the womb as completely helpless individuals, unlike animals such as horses and giraffes who have to stand and run within minutes of birth. It is often thought that a human baby is born too early, due to the size of the human head descending through the pelvis; any longer in the womb would make this passage impossible. To survive the baby has to rely upon an adult, usually the mother, for all their personal needs, feeding, cleaning and protection.

It is usual that in the first year of life the relationship between the mother and the baby grows close and strong. They become very familiar with each other and learn quickly when there are changes of mood and behaviour which may indicate that something is wrong. Consequently, parents have a key role to play in identifying when their child is finding something difficult to achieve. They are alert to signs of stress and anxiety, and such informal assessment and observation is probably the most important indicator of a child at risk of an IPD, and also of their particular strengths and weaknesses. Parents are therefore a vital part of any assessment, identification and intervention.

A child's home learning environment and the quality of parental engagement with them have been shown to be a key element in the development of resilience and a child's self-concept (Sroufe et al., 2005). Shaywitz (2005) reiterates this as the following quotation shows:

> Behind the success of every disabled child is a passionately committed, intensely engaged, and totally empowered parent, usually but not always the child's mother.
>
> (Shaywitz, 2005, p. 9)

Shaywitz (2005) also talks about the active and passive parent. The passive parent she cites as the one who want to 'wait and see', the one who thinks that their child's difficulties will all come right in the end. On the other side is the active parent, who actively seeks answers and searches tirelessly for explanations and understanding, sifting through the new research and championing their child's support needs.

> A child who has such a champion will not only succeed academically but will maintain his sense of self and the possibilities for a happy future.
>
> (Shaywitz, 2005, p. 174)

The problem for such an active parent is that there are so many approaches out there, so much research (some rigorous and some less so) that, particularly for the non-specialist, it can make it seem as though they are being bombarded with information and they do not know which to believe and which direction to take.

> An unwavering commitment to the intrinsic value of a child with dyslexia is essential ... All dyslexics who have become successful by any account share in common the unfailing love and support of their parents or occasionally, a teacher or a spouse.
>
> (Shaywitz, 2005, p. 309)

Cultural expectations

Reid (2016) suggests that the ability to read a language could be the defining element of a society and its culture. This is particularly so in the multi-cultural society of the UK today. The need for schools and teachers to understand the culture of the families of the children in their care ensures that this is a two-way conduit of communication between schools and families. Reid (2016) also believes that only when schools really understand the children's home cultures can they enable learning to take place, because learning can only occur when we start to build on prior learning, on established memories and on what we already know, so that we can advance from the known into the unknown. Welcoming diversity as a rich learning resource thereby becomes a truly positive and inclusive environment.

We know that dyslexia transcends all races and cultures, but Morgan and Klein (2000) showed that teachers are often reluctant to identify dyslexia in those for whom English is not their first language, preferring to think that it is a spoken language barrier that is to blame for the difficulties experienced. It is likely that when English is not their first language that this results in a misdiagnosis of IPDs in both children and adults. Dyslexia is no doubt overlooked when teachers and assessors feel that they have other difficulties to overcome, which could result in their failure to achieve, such as alternative cultures, bi/multilingualism, emotional difficulties, perhaps caused by displacement and fear (such as might be experienced by refugee children), limited English language skills and restricted vocabulary or limited social skills. It can certainly be hard to distinguish the origins of such difficulties and this can cause a major mismatch between their potential ability and the visible standard of their work.

A socio-cultural view of dyslexia emphasises the role of the parent, families, teachers and more experienced others, to support a child's learning in the Vygotskian tradition of ZPD (Zone of Proximal Development). From the moment of birth, each individual comes to the world with ever increasing amounts of knowledge and experience which is unique to their environment and conceptualisation. This shared experience of the world is what instigates our worldview and hence an ever evolving culture. This cultural experience is passed from one generation to another and families are often so immersed in their culture that the importance of passing this on to their children ensures that their beliefs and values define that particular culture. This sharing of culture usually starts with the sharing of language and symbolism, affording a particular identity to that culture. This can unintentionally become a problem if the culture of the home learning environment is different to that of the school or employment. Wearmouth (2002) showed that teachers frequently saw bi/multilingualism as a problem which offered a deficit view of families; this is perverse when the UK has been shown to be the most monolingual country in Europe. Burge et al. (2013) showed that only 64.8% of the residents of the UK were able to communicate in a second language, compared to 98% of the residents of Poland; this has the potential to significantly harm our international economy and multilingualism needs to be celebrated rather than castigated.

One advantage of the familial aspect of this condition is that many children with an IPD have parents who also have an IPD: they can often identify with the difficulties that their child is experiencing. However, in some families the child identified is the only one, and non-dyslexic parents often find it hard to empathise with the struggles that their child is facing. It is likely that they must first gain the knowledge before they can be a true advocate for their child in school and in life. Morgan and Klein (2000) suggest that in some cultures it is seen as shameful to admit that a child has any type of disability or difficulty and they prefer to blame language barriers or immigration status.

Many children will arrive at school from rich literary cultures, but these cultures may be very different from the one they will experience in school. This is exacerbated when the home language is also different from the school.

> Unfamiliarity with local culture, customs and language on entering school can result in complete bewilderment and an inability to understand the expectations and norms of the literacy curriculum.
> (Berryman and Wearmouth, 2009, p. 342)

Dyslexia Friendly Schools

The British Dyslexia Association's (BDA) Dyslexia Friendly Schools initiative was set up in 1999. This emphasised the need for a close partnership with parents by building communication with parents, many of whom will be feeling angry and frustrated by the likely delays in identification and support for their child. This initiative aims to build parental confidence, improve relationships with teachers and parents, and increase collaboration between parents and schools by engaging with those parents and listening to their points of view and acting upon them. In this way trust is engendered and partnerships formed to encourage the parents and their children to feel secure enough to consult with, and confide in, their teachers and schools by respecting parents and their potential contributions.

Families

As a teacher for many years, I frequently heard the words *You're the teacher ... you teach him!* but this negates and undervalues the role of families to learning. Families are the child's first and foremost teachers, certainly when it comes to social and emotional learning. It is vital that all children feel that their family, including their extended family, understand and support them. This is particularly important for children with any sort of learning difference. This requires considerable investment on the part of the family, of time, money and knowledge. However, it is important that families strike a balance between being supportive and becoming over-anxious, pressurising and over-bearing.

There is little doubt that the identification of dyslexia in a child will bring immense strains to a family. Morgan and Klein (2000) cite a number of factors which may influence the degree of that stress:

1. The age at which the individual is identified – this could be as a child or as an adult.
2. The nature and degree of intervention and support in place.
3. The amount of what Morgan and Klein (2000) described as 'excess baggage' which has accumulated within the family prior to the identification ... For example, how much do they know about dyslexia? ... Have relationships in the family already broken down? ... Has there already been a loss of self-esteem? ... Do the family regard it as a stigma?
4. The severity of the manifestations of the condition.
5. Cultural expectations.
6. The number of other family members affected, and the child's birth position within that family.

The importance of self-image to someone with an IPD is a key factor in the support that children get from their parents. Those with a positive self-image tend to come from homes that regard them as significant and interesting in their own right, so they are listened to and respected. These homes are likely to have parents with reasonable and consistent expectations of their child's ability to succeed. However, it is not just parents that have this influence, but all family members, intergenerational and other significant adults, such as teachers, teaching assistants, play workers, child carers etc. Children quickly become aware of the levels of expectation that significant adults have of them and if they feel that their achievements do not match these expectations, that is when they experience a sense of failure. Children are very adept at identifying and assessing the levels of expectation from their important adults.

It is important however, to realise that a final recognition that the family member does have a particular problem – is not just stupid or lazy or recalcitrant – can also come as an immense relief to a family, providing an explanation for the behaviour that has caused so much frustration and anger in the family.

REFLECT ON THIS

In a quiet moment consider the following questions:

1. What problems can you remember having at school and why?
2. Was there anyone particularly helpful in overcoming these problems?
3. What do you think it was that made the help so positive?
4. Was home a positive experience for you and why?
5. How did your home life and support provide you with a firm base to go forward in life?
6. Was there anyone in your life that you could talk to in confidence, and why did you feel that you could talk to them?

Parenting a child is probably the most important thing that an adult will ever have to do, and parenting a child who does not quite fit the norm is probably the most challenging. There is no such thing as a 'perfect' parent, so being a parent is really just about doing your best, taking advice and championing the cause for your child. Parents are likely to experience every emotion and often at their extremes: love/hate, pride/shame, joy/despair, rage/calm, grief/hope, confusion/certainty etc. As a consequence, any behaviour in their child that they do not understand or is out of the ordinary can be scary and confusing, and can lead parents to reflect upon their own parenting skills. Are they doing it right? Are they any good as a parent? Even simple everyday events can become problems, helping their child to walk, organising their routines, tidying up, etc. This can be further exacerbated when parents themselves have little self-confidence, have low self-esteem and maybe struggle themselves with reading, information processing, memory, organisation etc.

Parents and families need to understand that what the child with dyslexia needs is a supportive environment and supportive adults need to show that they:

1. Recognise and value what the child does and says.
2. Try to understand what the child is feeling.
3. Demonstrate interest in the child.
4. Actively listen to the child and acknowledge what they say and think.
5. Believe in the child's ability to achieve, even when it is hard.
6. Understand that time is their most valuable gift.
7. Accept and respect the child for the unique individual that they are.
8. Recognise the need to get help and take advice when necessary.
9. Maintain open and honest communication.

> The parents of children with specific learning difficulties (dyslexia) frequently experience considerable problems in obtaining from LEAs the special educational provision that they consider their children need. One of the consequences of LMS [local management of schools] is that all educational activities will be costed. The legal obligation on LEAs and schools to provide resources for the assessment and alleviation of specific learning difficulties (dyslexia) are likely to lead to considerably more legal action pressure groups backing disaffected parents.
> (Pumfrey and Reason, 1991, p. 49)

Despite this, in 2019, the All-Party Parliamentary Group (APPG) showed that 95% of parents felt ill equipped to support their children with dyslexia, and nearly half of them spent over £1,000 per year directly related to supporting their child. This same report showed that over 58% of their children avoided discussing their difficulties and 82% said that their children were embarrassed by their dyslexia and tried to hide their difficulties.

What about me?

The siblings of an individual with an IPD can also experience anxiety and stress. Attention given to the child with dyslexia can mean parents unintentionally overlook the particular needs of the other siblings. In some cases, the brothers and sisters may feel a responsibility for their dyslexic sibling, particularly in school, where they may, for example, feel the need to come to the aid of a bullied sibling, or may feel proud of their achievements. This may, on the surface, seem to a parent to be a very positive reaction, but could in fact be a precursor to the siblings' own difficulties, and, by drawing attention to the differences between siblings, can give rise to all kinds of inter-sibling rivalry, even leading potentially to serious aggression. Negatively, the sibling may also feel embarrassed by how the dyslexic brother or sister behaves in school and around their peers and also about their lower level of achievement. In the eyes of the non-dyslexic children, parents may appear to spend more time and energy with the dyslexic sibling, give more help with their homework, spend more time with them at appointments with psychologists and the school. They may also have many unanswered questions such as *Have I got this condition? Can I catch it?* etc. At times they may feel resentful and angry towards the dyslexic sibling, when parents give the dyslexic child fewer roles and responsibilities in the home, especially if they have difficulties with memory, following instructions, etc. This can bring about feelings of guilt and jealousy, as the dyslexic sibling appears, even to their parents, to be getting more time spent on them, more attention and even more money spent on computers, other gadgets and additional teaching. This may cause them to behave badly in an attempt to get the parental attention they feel they deserve. Factors that can affect this are:

- The age of the child and their siblings
- The age gap between the siblings
- Gender differences
- Family size.

Often the child with an IPD will be compared to other children in the family *your big sister was so much better at ... than you!* or *work hard and you can be top of the class, just like your brother.* This can be even more distressing when the sibling is younger, so giving rise to many inter-sibling rivalries, even aggressive incidents.

Peer group

A peer group can have a profound influence upon an individual at any point in their lives, but particularly in their formative school years. Many of those that I interviewed for this book described feelings of isolation and loneliness and of not having friends at school, often resulting in social exclusion and a very unhappy time. This in turn can be what can turn a child, desperate to make friends and be in with the peer group, into the class clown, the one who does things that no one else dares to do, the one who shouts back at the teacher, throws things across the room, etc. Although the peer group are shocked by this behaviour, there is also a small part that admires their classmate for doing something they do not quite dare to do themselves. Desperate attempts to make friends and ingratiate themselves with the peer group, this is the child who brings cigarettes into school, alcohol, drugs and other illicit items to share with and sell to the other children. Discovery only enhances the title of naughty, uncontrollable, dangerous, etc., but it also earns the bearer a kudos that they cannot achieve in the academic environment, and they find themselves surrounded by pseudo-friends and admirers who want to be seen with them.

Interview

John, now in his fifties, recalls bitterly his time in school:

> My parents had a newspaper shop and sold cigarettes and tobacco, I used to sneak down from our flat above the shop and steal a packet of cigarettes. The next day I would take them into school and sell them at 50p each. I always had lots of takers and people would seek me out, and hang around with me to get the odd freebie. At the time I thought they were my friends but as I look back, I realise that this was not so and when the school found out and suspended me these, so-called friends, were nowhere to be seen. It caused a lot of trouble with my family, who at first could not believe that I had done this. They wanted to believe the best in me, but I now see that I brought a lot of heartache and disgrace to my family.

Learned helplessness

Learned helplessness is a phenomenon which occurs when we believe (not necessarily correctly) that we have no way out of a difficult situation, when we relinquish the idea of control and our ability to control what is happening to us. Seligman (1998) proposed this idea after putting animals, usually dogs and rats, into electrified boxes and subjecting them to electric shocks. Similar experiments were later used with humans, using loud noises rather than electric shocks. What Seligman (1998) found was that if the subject believed that nothing could be done about their circumstances, they would eventually give up trying to escape the situation. Seligman believes that we are not born to be so accepting of an adverse situation, so it must be a learned or conditioned response. Abramson et al. (1978) agrees with Seligman and subdivides this phenomenon into two types:

1 Universal helplessness: this is where individuals believe that nothing can be done about the situation that they are in.
2 Personal helplessness: the individual believes that something could be done about their situation, but they have no control over it, control is with others who are not (for whatever reason) asserting that control.

In both cases the individual believes that there is no point in trying to seek a way out to relieve the despair, hence the possible development of low self-esteem, poor motivation and even depression.

Seligman (1998) believed that it is not helpful to cushion a child from all failure, and it is important for them to experience an element of failure before they can really appreciate the feelings of success. Having to work at something with an equal weight of success and failure is a vital part of the holistic development of the child. Seligman (1998) believed that we need to set realistic goals for children to enable achievement, not every time, but on enough occasions to develop what he called an *accurate optimism* (p. 298).

Talking to individuals with dyslexia over the years, parents and families clearly feature very highly in their ability to cope with the difficulties of living in a non-dyslexic world. However, becoming too dependent on others could possibly induce learned helplessness, the idea that they cannot cope alone without that help and support. Parents, families and peers can help by suggesting strategies to enable the individual with dyslexia to manage alone and achieve success by not fearing failure, rather embracing it and achieving independence. This takes patience and trust which is something that most parents, families, peers and those close to us often have in abundance.

Chapter reflections

What you have read in this chapter demonstrates the implications of living with someone with an IPD, socially, emotionally and financially. The whole issue of the balance of nature versus nurture, or inheritance versus the environment, is highly controversial, but dyslexia and other IPDs do seem to run in families; it is highly unlikely that we will ever be able to determine exactly how much of this is due to nature and how much to nurture. We know that genes provide the blueprint for our existence, but the interplay between our genes and the environment, which give rise to gene expression or epigenesis, is a very new area of research. It is increasingly seen as a vital factor in how humans develop. Children are completely dependent upon parents and adults for the foods they eat, the exercise they take, sleep patterns, lifestyle, where they live, stress levels and even the levels of drugs and alcohol in their lives. All these, and more, can influence the chemicals within the body that switch on or switch off that gene expression.

REFLECT ON THIS

With a friend or colleague reflect upon the following two questions:

1   How important do you think it is to continue the research to determine the balance of nature versus nurture in child development?
2   Do you believe that the prenatal stage of the development of a child is determined by nature or nurture and why?

In order to best help a child who has an IPD there needs to be intense communication and negotiation between families and schools, but each will have their own competing priorities, and it may be that in the future some form of mediation service needs to be implemented. Parents and families are perhaps best placed to see the person as a whole individual, not just a schoolchild or a working colleague, but to see not only the challenges, but also the many things that they can achieve and do well. When this works well, they can act as a conduit between the individual with an IPD and the school or employer, helping them to organise, listen and celebrate the unique successes, and potentially the very positive contribution that this person can make to society.

The next chapter examines the impact of an IPD to the health and mental health of an individual and considers the effects upon the health services in this country, of treating the health conditions which often become an unwanted bi-product of an IPD.

Further reading

Amira, A, Raufl, A, Akmar, MI, Balakrishnan, V and Harunal, K (2018) Dyslexic children: the need for parents' awareness. *Journal of Education and Human Development* 7(2): 91–99. https://www.researchgate.net/publication/326913779_Dyslexic_Children_The_Need_for_Parents_Awareness/download (accessed 20.11.19).

The focus of this research paper is upon parents in Malaysia who have children with dyslexia. Despite the many cultural differences between Malaysia and the UK, it has a great deal to tell us of the struggles that parents have to be an effective advocate for their child. It emphasises the need for parental awareness of the condition, and suggests that it is *imperative in ensuring sustainable development of the children*. The paper also emphasises the importance of early identification and intervention to the well-being of both the child and parent. The paper calls for more knowledge for parents and better support systems to aid the families.

References

Abramson, LY, Seligman, ME and Teasdale, JD (1978) Learned helplessness in humans: critique and reformulation. *Journal of Abnormal Psychology*, 87(1): 49–74.

All-Party Parliamentary Group for Dyslexia and other SpLDs (APPG) *The Human Cost of Dyslexia: The Emotional and Psychological Impact of Poorly Supported Dyslexia*. BDA. www.bdadyslexia.org.uk/about/all-party-parliamentary-group-dyslexia-and-spld-appg (accessed 20. 11. 19).

Amira, A, Raufl, A, Akmar, MI, Balakrishnan, V and Harunal, K (2018) Dyslexic children: the need for parents' awareness. *Journal of Education and Human Development* 7(2): 91–99. https://www.researchgate.net/publication/326913779_Dyslexic_Children_The_Need_for_Parents_Awareness/download (accessed 20. 11. 19).

Berryman, M and Wearmouth, J (2009) Responsive approaches to literacy within cultural contexts. In Reid, G (2009) (ed) *The Routledge Companion to Dyslexia*. Abingdon: Routledge.

Burge, B, Ager, R, Cook, R, Cunningham, R, Morrison, J, Weaving, H and Wheater, R (2013) *European Survey on Language Competencies: Language Proficiency in England*. London: DfE.

Department for Education and Department of Health (2015) *Special Educational Needs and Disability Code of Practice: 0 to 25 Years*. https://www.gov.uk/government/publications/send-code-of-practice-0-to-25 (accessed 20. 11. 19).

Foss, B (2016) *The Dyslexia Empowerment Plan: Blueprint for Renewing Your Child's Confidence and Love of Learning*. New York: Ballantine Books.

Ghouri, S (1998) Mum's too afraid to ask. *Times Educational Supplement*, 4th September.

Hartas, D (2006) *Dyslexia in the Early Years: A Practical Guide to Teaching and Learning*. Oxon: Routledge.

Morgan, E and Klein, C (2000) *The Dyslexic Adult in a Non-Dyslexic World*. London: Whurr Publications.

Nosek, K (1997) *Dyslexia in Adults: Taking Charge of Your Life*. Maryland, USA: Taylor Trade Publishing.

Pumfrey, P and Reason, R (1991) *Specific Learning Difficulties (Dyslexia) Challenges and Responses*. London: Routledge.

Reid, G (2016) *Dyslexia: A Practitioner's Handbook*. Chichester: Wiley.

Seligman, MEP (1998) The prediction and prevention of depression. In *The Science of Clinical Psychology: Accomplishments and Future Directions*. Washington DC: American Psychological Association.

Shaywitz, S (2005) *Overcoming Dyslexia*. New York: Vintage Books.

Sroufe, LA, Egland, B, Carlson, EA and Collins, WA (2005) *The Development of the Person: The Minnesota Study of Risk and Adaptation from Birth to Adulthood*. New York: Guilford.

Wearmouth, J (2002) The role of the learning support coordinator: addressing the challenges. In Reid, G and Wearmouth, J (eds), *Dyslexia and Literacy*. Chichester: John Wiley.

4 Health and mental health

> Don't let your struggle become your identity
> (Thought to be attributed to Ralston Bowles [1952–date],
> American singer/songwriter)

Introduction

This chapter will examine how some people clearly have more difficulty than others coping with the social and emotional strains of living with information processing differences (IPDs), and how this can, at times, develop into physical and mental health conditions such as psychosomatic conditions, depression, anxiety and even suicidal thoughts.

Research by Willcutt and Gaffney-Brown (2004) indicated that as many as 40% of people with dyslexia suffer from depression and other related anxiety disorders, as opposed to 25% in the general population in the UK (Mind, 2013). There would appear to be no evidence that dyslexia is caused by such mental health issues, so it is possible that dyslexia and IPDs are in some way a trigger for such mental health conditions. With the numbers involved it is vital that those working in the health services have a comprehensive understanding of how IPDs can impact the lives of their patients, and how their ability to help, both children and adults with IPDs, can be severely compromised if they are not recognised and understood.

Inside and out

Living with a constant barrage of criticism and perceived failure is undoubtably hard, and many of the interviews conducted for this book intimated just that, especially during the school years, where there is constant assessment and expectation. Many who live with an IPD manage to overcome this and build a tough exterior to the constant condemnation and disapproval; they develop resilience in their lives. However, for some this does not work, and they find this constant negativity too threatening and intimidating. A review of the relevant literature by Boyes et al. (2016) suggests that there is a strong correlation between children with reading difficulties and later mental health problems, although they do admit that the numbers vary between studies, and what is less clear is why that correlation exists. This study divides the problem into what they call internalised or emotional difficulties (anxiety, depression, psychosomatic complaints, withdrawal, etc); these are issues within the self, and external or behavioural difficulties (conduct disorder, conflict with others, anger, aggression, rule breaking behaviours, etc). Interestingly a Norwegian study by Dahle and Knivsberg (2015) showed a higher detection and identification rate of externalised symptoms than internalised, particularly by teachers, compared to parents who were more likely to identify the internalised symptoms.

Edwards (1994) suggests that children, with what are referred to in this study as Specific Learning Difficulties (SpLDs), are more sensitive to criticism than those without. This idea is reiterated by Riddick (2010), but a number of questions arise from such a premise: firstly are these children already genetically pre-disposed to over-sensitivity, in other words this could be a co-occurring condition with an IPD. Secondly, is the question of the reality behind the idea that individuals identified with an IPD receive more criticism; it could simply be a perceptual issue. Research by Edwards (1994) did appear to show that children with dyslexia received more negative comments on their work in school from teachers than those without (the teachers justified this by saying that it was important feedback to their pupils). It also appeared that in this research the children focused more on the negative comments than the positive (of which there was much). It would seem, in this case, that perception and reality were interacting with each other to produce a feeling of unfairness and possibly stress. Riddick (2010) suggests that this is a cyclical process, so the more criticism received the more negative the thoughts and the more likely that feelings of inadequacy, anxiety and depression will occur, perhaps resulting in over-sensitivity to further criticism (Figure 4.1).

Elmer (2001) concluded that the way that some individuals respond to negative feedback differs from others, some appear able to ignore it, but what is less certain is why this might be. Elmer (2001) points to a possible genetic connection but does not rule out a strong environmental element. The difficulty of this nature versus nurture debate is proving it, and research to do so is unlikely to be ethically acceptable and would be methodologically extremely difficult.

A spoonful of sugar

Stress is like that spoonful of sugar that helps the medicine go down – too much sugar and there is a risk of overweight and obesity, and all the accompanying health issues that are discussed repeatedly in the newspapers. Too little sugar and the medicine is unpalatable and not ingested, resulting in a plethora of health issues. Too much stress can lead to anxiety and depression and worse, too little stress and there is no motivation to learn or to take on

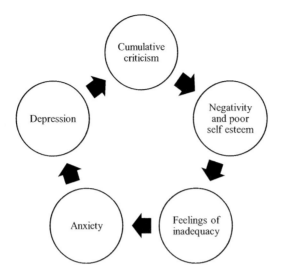

Figure 4.1 Cyclical process of criticism leading to depression

new challenges. Reid (2017) agrees with Elmer (2001) and Edwards (1994) that some people may be more prone to the negative effects of stress than others, but believes that the triggers for stress are likely to be different from one individual to another. What for one person is a damaging start to a downward spiral is to another just of mild concern and of no consequence. Reid (2017) points out that not only are the triggers for stress likely to be different from one individual to another, but age and stage of development will also influence what we stress about. What can be a cause of concern for a small child (a best friend not wanting them to play with them) is likely to be different from the adolescent (impending GCSEs, spots and acne making them less desirable), to the adult (paying the rent/mortgage, etc). For this reason, it is important that employers, teachers and parents take stress very seriously, with an understanding and awareness of its potential for positive motivation, as well as possible damage, to achieve the right balance of realistic expectation and ambition for that individual.

Stress is the body's natural response to keeping it safe from something either physical, such as getting too close to a cliff edge, or something psychological, such as taking an important exam or knowing that you are going to be asked to read in front of a group of other individuals. Alexandre-Passe (2015a) describes stress as an attempt to protect our body from what he calls stress triggers. He also talks about 'good' stress and 'bad' stress. Good stress, he suggests, allows us to feel empowered and able to overcome all that comes our way. Bad stress produces indecision and disempowerment, and can be linked to smoking, poor eating habits, anorexia, alcohol and substance abuse, susceptibility to infections such as colds and flu, depression, insomnia, heart disease and even cancer. For these triggers to produce such a reaction, the part of the brain called the amygdala must make connections between a particular circumstance and its possible consequences. When an individual feels in control of a situation, this stress reaction can prove to be very positive, alerting the body to the circumstance, keeping us 'on our toes' and allowing problem solving to overcome the adverse situation. However, some triggers will cause the body to feel out of control, that there is no way of preventing the negative outcome, and this then becomes harmful stress.

When worries become long term then chronic stress can occur, which is difficult to overcome. Those with dyslexia often find themselves with chronic stress, being constantly on high alert to the possibility of making errors or 'showing themselves up' in public, for others to ridicule. This can result in isolating themselves from others, avoiding the social situations which will induce the triggers, to prevent the possibility of these very public errors. Thomson (1996) talks about two opposing reactions to the stress of dyslexia in school aged children, internalising and externalising symptoms: some will withdraw from the situation which can result in trembling, sweating, refusal to integrate, etc. The second is an overreaction, resulting in the 'class clown', the 'I don't care' attitude, even aggression and other overtly poor behaviour. Thus, chronic stress and chronic anxiety can extend to all aspects of life both physical and mental, and often results in unhappiness and misery.

Anxiety

Anxiety is what happens when the individual perceives that there will be a stress trigger, before it happens (Alexandre-Passe, 2015a). In simple terms, this is worrying about what *might* happen, as opposed to stress, which is a reaction to what *is* happening at the time.

> It is the difference between perceived and present stressors that differentiates anxiety from fear.
> (Alexander-Passe, 2015a, p. 121)

Anxiety can manifest itself in many different ways, ranging from nail biting and nervous habits to post traumatic stress disorder. The NHS website (NHS, 2019) offers a list of possible physical symptoms associated with anxiety:

- Dizziness
- Tiredness and insomnia
- Palpitations
- Aches and pains
- Shaking
- Dry mouth
- Unable to breath normally
- Sweating

- Stomach disorders
- Vomiting and nausea
- Headaches
- Pins and needles in the extremities.

For the individual with an IPD this can be brought on by the anticipated fear of failure and of making the wrong decisions, and by the fear of being seen as a disappointment to family, schools and employers. This can in turn result in the individual avoiding particular areas that induce those feelings of anxiety, such as avoiding reading (particularly reading aloud), writing, social activities, sports and relationships, for fear of being seen as stupid or lazy.

> To some, stress is a challenge to overcome, whereas to others it is too much of a challenge, leading to an emotional overload of distress/panic. Thus, it is personally constructed and hard to measure.
> (Alexander-Passe, 2015a)

Interview

John, now retired, was a hospital doctor.

> I came from a family who, when I reflect back, were probably all dyslexic – at least most of them – so some of the more bizarre experiences that I had felt very 'normal'.
>
> School was a nightmare, I was always in trouble, and I really could not read with any level of fluency until I was nine or 10 years old. I'm not sure how I ended up in the medical profession, as I hate reading even today. Everyone was amazed when I passed my 11+ and went to a grammar school. Despite taking three attempts to get English O-level, I finally achieved and got accepted for medical school. I never told anyone that I was dyslexic, and, as a student, would never let anyone read my notes, as I was so ashamed of my scrawny handwriting and even more bizarre spelling. I relied heavily on friends and fellow students to help me, and somehow they never guessed my problem (well I don't think so), but recognised that I did not come out with them to parties, instead I worked hard, often throughout the night when it was quiet and peaceful, to enable me to learn the anatomical terms and Latin names for diseases and conditions.
>
> When I started work in the hospital, my biggest problem was time management. Doctors work strictly to timed periods with the patients, and I had to ask the nurses to keep me on track. It was the nurses who often wrote up notes for me to ensure that I had it right, and there were certain things that I would never volunteer to do. At first, I didn't tell them about my dyslexia, but in the end, I realise that they could support me, and were happy to do so. I always checked and double checked all my decisions and all my reports; I knew what I wanted to say but often could not think how to spell it.

I think if I had told anyone when I went from my initial interviews, I would never have got the jobs and probably would never have become a doctor, which is really what I am passionate about.

Psychosomatic disorders

In a study by Riddick (2010), mothers of children who had been identified with dyslexia were asked about whether they had seen any physical effects which impacted their children living with dyslexia. A number of common features to their responses were identified:

- Bedwetting
- Tantrums
- Sleep disturbances
- Anger
- Stammering
- Excessive need for comfort items such as blankets, soft toys, etc.
- Vomiting
- Eating disorders
- Unexplained aches and pains.

Although stress is usually seen as an issue involving the working of the brain, it can also trigger profound physical reactions or psychosomatic conditions, in which the mind and body interact negatively as chemicals such as adrenaline/epinephrine flood the body, triggering a fight or flight response: *do I run away from this attacker with a knife, or do I face up to him?* Such chemical changes can produce increased heart pumping, high blood pressure, and changes in metabolic rate and blood glucose concentrations (Alexander-Passe, 2015a). On a more positive note, chemical changes such as these are vital for our safety and protection, highlighting our ability to make decisions quickly and appropriately; however, an over-production of such chemicals, or more prolonged production, can have the reverse effect by creating feelings of confusion and panic, thereby possibly making decision making more difficult, inappropriate and extreme. The balance between stress that is 'normal' and too much stress is a fine line, probably dependent upon age, maturity, previous life experiences, levels of resilience and the amount of support.

Some physical conditions are more prone to being brought on by stress and anxiety, for example eczema, psoriasis, stomach ulcers, high blood pressure, heart disease and chest pains. Most people have experienced this in a mild way when the mind produces physical symptoms, for example, when sitting important exams or attending an interview, when the heart starts to race, nausea, sweaty palms, butterflies in the stomach and shaking can occur. These are not imagined symptoms, they are very real to the person involved, brought on by the stress hormones /chemicals. Edwards (1994) also reported incidents of psychosomatic pain from her case studies of eight students, all identified with dyslexia, when three of the eight reported such symptoms.

Depression

According to the National Health Service website (NHS, 2019), depression is about a persistent feeling of sadness and helplessness. The emphasis here is upon the word 'persistent': inevitably we all have days when we feel down in the dumps and fed up, but we can usually attribute this to a particular issue in our lives at the time. Depression can also be linked to associated physical conditions such as tiredness, lack of appetite, poor sex drive, and aches and pains. However, clinical depression is a very real and potentially dangerous chronic health condition, sometimes lasting days, weeks, months and even years. Unfortunately, despite this being a serious medical condition, the way the word *depression* has entered our lexicon means that it is used repeatedly in general conversation to mean feeling 'fed up', or moody, implying a condition of not much consequence that is easy to lift.

Depression can be seen on a graduated scale ranging from very mild and transitionary to severe, persistent and serious (Figure 4.2).

According to the NHS (2019), depression probably affects about 10% of the population in the UK at some point in their lives, so it can be regarded as a relatively common condition with approximately 4% of children under the age of sixteen experiencing some level of depression.

Those who suffer from depression describe some of the symptoms:

- Constant low mood and personality changes
- Feelings of helplessness, despair and anxiety
- Low self-esteem
- Frequently tearful
- Feeling irrationally guilty
- Irritability and loss of sociability
- Sleep problems
- Lacking motivation and concentration
- Memory impairments and mental confusion
- Poor decision making
- Unhappy
- Altered speech patterns
- Poor or voracious appetite with frequent digestive problems

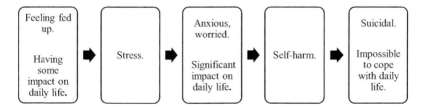

Figure 4.2 Graduated scale of depression

- Constipation
- Changes to menstrual cycle
- Headaches
- Self-harming
- Suicide or suicidal thoughts.

According to Scott (2004), there is a fundamental gender split in the way that males and females experience depression. Her research showed that males are more likely to externalise their frustrations into aggression and overtly bad behaviour, whereas females are more likely to withdraw, eventually internalising their feelings and lapsing into depression. Interestingly research by Shaywitz (2005) indicated a similar gender difference; she suggests that this is one reason why it has always been perceived that there are more male children with dyslexia than females. However, she suggests that more males are *identified* because their behaviour is more overt and difficult to deal with in a classroom situation, so they are more likely to be sent for assessment than the quieter, more retiring and withdrawn girls, thereby giving the impression of an imbalance in the gender split.

Scott (2004) acknowledges that whilst most individuals with dyslexia and IPDs will not experience depression, there is a higher proportion than would be expected in the rest of the population. This she suggests is a natural consequence of experiencing years of feeling a failure.

Self-harm

Scott (2004) suggests that there is a high correlation between dyslexia and drugs and alcohol abuse, with addictions to tobacco, cocaine, marijuana, ecstasy and anti-depressants. Eating disorders such as binge eating, anorexia and bulimia also correlate highly with dyslexia, as does cutting, punching, pinching and deliberately breaking bones or ingesting toxic substances. All of these appear to be an attempt, on behalf of the individual, to regain some level of personal control over their lives.

Hawton et al. (2002) undertook a large, self-reporting study, of 4,000 15–16-year olds and showed that 6.9% had engaged in self-harming activities, with as many as 12.6% of these leading to hospital admissions. This is likely to be a conservative estimate as self-harming is often a secretive and covert activity which may not be reported.

Unfortunately, dyslexia and substance abuse is an area which is woefully short of reliable empirical research, but Scott (2004) suggests that 60% of dyslexic individuals, in her research, also declared that they drank alcohol to overcome anxiety. She found a high correlation between drug and alcohol abuse and dyslexia, both in children (some as young as thirteen), and adults. She claims that health and education professionals often try to treat the symptoms of such abuse, rather than looking beneath this at the underlying and root causes.

The average cost of someone presenting to hospital for self-harm (either poisoning or injury) is estimated by Tsiachristas et al. (2017) at £809 per patient; on this estimate of the numbers of self-harmers, it could be costing the National Health Service up to £162 million per annum, which is money which could possibly be better diverted to prevention of self-harm, rather than applying a sticking plaster after the event.

Suicide and suicidal thoughts

For some the pain and negativity that they feel when coping every day with an IPD is too great, and research by Riddick (2010) showed some mothers who said that their children wanted to kill themselves, rather than live for the rest of their lives with dyslexia. Links between dyslexia and suicide are well documented (Henderson and Thompson 2016), with attempts by school aged children increasing in term time and decreasing in the holidays. However, the *real* number of suicide attempts and those experiencing suicidal thoughts may never be known as they are usually not disclosed and remain private to the individual, not even shared with their family.

In a study by Alexander-Passe (2015b), he claims that as adults those with dyslexia,

> camouflage their difficulties with advanced coping strategies, so a sense of normality can be projected.
> (Alexander-Passe, 2015b)

They do this by creating a *secondary persona* or a front to the world, disguising their difficulties with a range of lies and half-truths: *I have forgotten my glasses, I haven't time to read this now* and such like. Like Henderson and Thompson (2016), Alexandre-Passe (2015b) also notes that there is a very close association between self-harm, suicidal thoughts, suicide and dyslexia, claiming this to be as high as a 40% correlation, but he also claims that this figure could be as high as 85%. However, as stated before, this is a figure which is extremely difficult to verify, and clearly there is the need for further more urgent and extensive research to be conducted in this area.

The film and television actress Susan Hampshire describes her experiences in her book:

> After I had been diagnosed as being dyslexic I couldn't be helped to overcome my dyslexia, because by that time I had got myself into such a state that I had a nervous breakdown ... I went catatonic and I was totally agoraphobic. I literally sat at home next to a radiator rocking back and forwards, for months and months ... when I tried to kill myself they put a care order on me and put me away in a special unit ... I was given all sorts of drugs.
> (Hampshire, 1990, p. 33)

In the compilation of interviews with people with dyslexia, Susan Hampshire (herself dyslexic) describes their battle with health and mental health. One interviewee, Rosemary, a beautician, recalls how she tried to commit suicide by slitting her wrists and eventually had a nervous breakdown at the age of sixteen. Rosemary was put on a real cocktail of drugs, some to help her to sleep, and some to keep her awake (Mogadon, Valium, etc). Clearly when dyslexia reaches these proportions the need for professional support, from the NHS, counsellors, therapists and social services, becomes imperative and literally a life and death situation.

Keeping a child in any form of care situation can, according to the National Audit Office (2014), cost as much as £200,000–300,000 per year, clearly making this a very expensive option for the tax payer. The NICE (National Institute for Health and Care Excellence) (2015) guidance estimates that each day spent in hospital costs the NHS £400. This, of course, fluctuates widely depending on the type of treatment. At a time when there are huge pressures on the resources of the NHS, patients who self-harm or make attempts upon their own life are only adding to the pressures unnecessarily and with the right support may never have needed to be in that situation.

Every year nearly one million people worldwide take their own life, every 40 seconds someone commits suicide and in the last forty-five years suicide rates have gone up by 60%. According to the Office for National Statistics (ONS) (2018), suicide is the second leading cause of death in 10–24-year-olds. In 2014 the ONS calculated that in England suicide had increased to 4,882 cases, and in Wales there are approximately 300 suicides a year, which is almost twice the number killed in road accidents; however, this is only the tip of the iceberg because there are probably many more unsuccessful and unreported attempts. Knapp et al. (2011) estimated that the cost of suicide in England was approximately £1.3 million each year based on a set of three criteria:

- The cost of services used by the individual up to and immediately after the suicide (GP, prescribed medication, counselling, funeral expenses, court costs, emergency services, insurance, etc.).
- The cost to society, such as time off work and loss of production.
- Human cost, such as the pain and grief for relatives and friends.

REFLECT ON THIS

Work with a friend or colleague and use a large sheet of paper to create a mind map of the possible feelings and difficulties that an individual with dyslexia may experience, related to their health and health care. One has already been started for you (Figure 4.3).

1   When you have filled the page look at it carefully, can you see any connections or contradictions between the items?
2   Do issues of gender, age or cultural heritage impact any of them?
3   Keep this mind map to refer to and perhaps add to later. Compare this to your own experiences.

Health and mental health 67

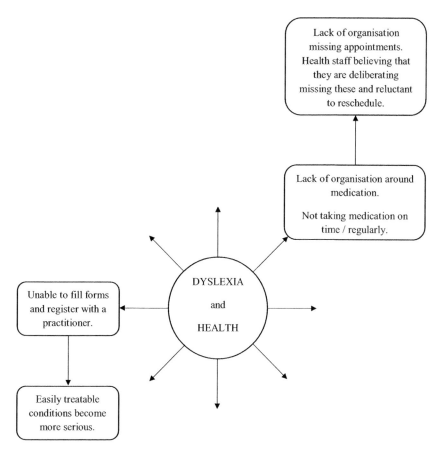

Figure 4.3 Mind map

Counselling

Counselling (and its many adaptations of cognitive programmes) is notoriously difficult to define, like dyslexia itself. However, it is certainly a verbal process of communication, and at its best it can provide emotional support and clarification in times of crisis, anxiety and unhappiness. Palmer et al. (1996), for the British Association for Counselling, describe the ideal relationship between client and counsellor as intense but dispassionate. The aim is to allow the client to 'let go' of their negative feelings in a neutral and unjudgmental manner through skilful and active listening, so that the client is helped to feel better about themselves. Any form of talking or listening process will be hugely time consuming, and by its very nature time involves a large financial consideration, so it is likely to be a long and expensive process for anyone feeling the emotional and mental health effects of dyslexia.

Health and care staff

It is not only those admitted to hospital who may have an IPD, and with prevalence levels for dyslexia in the general community being so high, it is highly probable that there will be medical staff who also work to cope with these conditions. The percentage of doctors and nurses with dyslexia is very difficult to measure, as like John in the interview earlier in this chapter, they tend to conceal their condition for fear of discrimination and prejudice. A study by Shaw and Anderson (2017) examined the experiences of medical students who had been identified as dyslexic. They concluded that with appropriate support, medical students with dyslexia could perform as well as those without; however, few asked for that support for fear of prejudicing their career or losing the confidence of their patients, so often there was no support available when they went out on their clinical placements. The exact number of qualified doctors identified with dyslexia is unknown, although a study by Newlands et al. (2014) estimates that up to 2% of UK doctors could be affected.

Morris and Turnball (2006) researched nursing students with dyslexia and showed that they were acutely aware of their own difficulties and were very concerned about the welfare of their patients, so checked their work repeatedly; many said that they referred to pocket electronic dictionaries, which they carried with them. This often made the time taken for a nurse with dyslexia to complete a task longer than their non-dyslexic colleagues.

According to Easton et al. (2013), low literacy (not necessarily dyslexia) can have a significant impact on access to the health services and the ability to self-manage health conditions resulting in generally poorer health outcomes. This study, whilst not specifically related to dyslexia, does indicate some of the very real problems that those with low levels of literacy can have with vital health related written information, and the often complex explanations and instructions that they receive from health professionals.

> Some communication difficulties were apparently perpetuated or exacerbated because participants limited their conversational engagement and used a variety of strategies to cover their low literacy that could send misleading signals to health professionals.
>
> (Easton et al., 2013)

This difficulty with communication is frequently brought about due to the stigma that patients feel concerning their levels of literacy, which appears to increase the likelihood of them self-excluding themselves from all manner of health services. Easton et al. (2013) recommended that the health service professional needed to have a greater awareness of the potential for their patients to have low literacy skills, and to better 'read' the signs that this could be the case. They needed to simplify the requirements for patients to read and write which were:

Non-judgemental (universal) literacy sensitive support to promote health care experiences and outcomes.

(Easton et al., 2013)

This study refers to this as 'health literacy' and shows that those with poor health literacy have less access to health and emergency services than the rest of the population, and chronic conditions such as asthma and diabetes are not managed as well, as the ability to manage a medication regime, particularly long-term preventative measures, is more difficult. This is particularly so for those with dyslexia who are also likely to have organisational difficulties and working memory lapses, which may mean that they do not always remember to carry their medication and have it available when needed. Such organisational lapses can also mean that patients with dyslexia miss or are late for appointments or arrive for their appointment unprepared, for example not bringing a requested urine sample or the right paperwork for an X ray request, etc.

Easton et al. (2013) showed that when a patient presented to the health care professional with spoken language difficulties, this was obvious, and support was usually put in place. However, when the difficulties were hidden, such as low literacy and dyslexia, the shame and stigma prevented patients from declaring this, and there was a low awareness by the health care staff of how to best identify and support their patient. Some patients in the study were diagnosed with stress, mental health problems, nervous breakdowns, eating disorders, panic attacks, but there was nothing to suggest that the doctor responsible for the diagnosis had explored the possibility of low literacy as a contributing factor. This important study appeared to show that there were likely to be difficulties for those with low literacy skills in four particular areas of health care:

1 Access and utilisation of health care
2 Patient and provider interaction
3 Self-care and medication administration
4 A reduced ability to obtain knowledge and understanding of their conditions.

There is a heavy reliance within the NHS on written material, with even the simplest procedure requiring form filling (even registering with a GP or dentist), and this is made even more difficult by the use of complex medical terminology and jargon that even those with highly tuned literacy skills find hard to understand.

REFLECT ON THIS

The following scenario is entirely fictious although I suspect that it is one played out quite regularly in our hospitals and health clinics across the country:

Sergio was bundled into the car by his boss having just fallen off a ladder at work. He felt OK but the boss insisted that he was checked out by a doctor. He was taken to the nearest hospital and his boss left him at the door before driving back to the building site to supervise the other workers. He asked Sergio if he would be OK on his own, but Sergio assured him that he was, and said that he would ring him when he was ready to return home.

Sergio walked straight into reception and asked the way to the accident and emergency department. The receptionist was very helpful and told him that he had come to the wrong department but told him to go through the double doors, turn left and follow the signs suspended from the ceiling indicating osteopathy and then turn left again when he would see the signs for A and E. Sergio smiled and walked off through the double doors but was unsure which was left and which right (he had already forgotten the instructions beyond here). His mum had always told him that he would 'write with his right', so he physically moved his right hand and pretended to hold a pencil ... this was what he always did when he was not sure.

There were so many signs above his head with words on them that meant nothing to him and he had never seen before. He carried on walking down the corridor with lots of people rushing past him who all seemed to know where they were going and how to get there, they seemed busy and confident. He probably looked a bit muddled so one nurse stopped and kindly asked him if he was lost and needed help, she directed him to the A and E department.

Once inside the busy section he presented himself to the receptionist, who after a little wait gave him a small electronic device and asked him to read the touch screen carefully and answer the questions. The receptionist did ask him whether he was familiar with a touch screen and Sergio nodded. However, the receptionist did not ask him whether he needed assistance to read the questions. Not wishing to look foolish when there were so many people around and a queue behind him, he took the device and stared at the screen for some time, but most of the questions meant nothing to him. He wrote his name and address and date of birth, but when asked whether he had eaten that day, or whether he also suffered from conditions such as diabetes or epilepsy, he was at a loss. Sergio could feel the stress rising in his stomach and pretended to write on the screen so that those around him would not think that there was a problem. After some time and other patients had come in and completed their survey, Sergio could stand it no longer and returned the device to the receptionist and walked out of the hospital without seeing a doctor.

1. How typical do you think this scenario might be?
2. How could Sergio's experience have been made more welcoming and less stressful?
3. What sort of training do you think should be essential for all front-line staff in health service establishments?

4   Potentially what negative impact could there be on Sergio, and others like him, who have been denied access to the sort of health care that most of us take for granted?
5   How likely do you think it is that Sergio and others like him, will try to access health care in the future?

Interview

On a more positive note was an interview conducted with Yvette, now semi-retired but a nurse in the NHS for many years.

> When I was in training, we were encouraged to view the patients as holistic beings and to take on board the whole person as they presented before us. This meant really listening to the patient, undertaking detailed observations of them (even if that was a snapshot). However, that takes time and, in the NHS today this is sometimes in short supply. I always checked that my patients were able to read any material that I gave them, and if I did suspect that they had any sort of reading or language difficulty would go through it with them. In the long run it saved time, as patents did not need to return at a later date with more acute symptoms, because they were not following instructions or did not understand the directions.

Yvette later worked as a school nurse:

> As a school nurse, I was able to build up my relationship with the children and their parents. Some of the children would come to me to read to me as I presented as a friendly and non-judgemental figure. I was acutely aware that letters home, concerning vaccinations or health checks, would often not be read, and if a parent did not attend an appointment or respond to the letters, it was probably not because they did not care, but more likely that they did not or could not read the letters. I would make an extra effort to talk to these parents directly and inform them of their appointments.

Chapter reflections

Although this chapter appears to focus upon some very negative aspects of dyslexia, it is also intended to indicate the positives, and this is a theme that will be followed in chapter eight of this book, where the idea that those with IPDs can bring something very positive to society will be explored. It is vital that those who feel in the depths of despair about their dyslexia, even if they do not at that stage recognise it as that, seek professional support and take control of their condition, to feel more empowered. Some of this chapter makes very grim reading, but it is also important to remember that not all individuals identified with dyslexia or an IPD will have any of the social and emotion difficulties discussed here. On a more positive note, some NHS Foundation Trusts are attempting to raise awareness of dyslexia in their staff, and some have even appointed Ambassadors for Dyslexia, to help to raise the profile of both colleagues and patients with an IPD. Several Trusts have also been involved with Dyslexia Awareness Week, organised by the British Dyslexia Association.

> Not surprisingly, participants advocated the simplification of written information, including signage, appointment letters and instructions for medicine-taking, as well as healthcare leaflets. They also suggested that their understanding of clinical information and advice could be much improved if healthcare professionals explained things in lay terms rather than using medical terminology and jargon.
>
> (Easton et al., 2013)

Talking to so many people with an IPD and their families, who are coping with this condition in their lives, it is clear that the most difficult time of life for those with IPD is during their time in schools and colleges, and the next chapter will attempt to show some of the flavour of this and to highlight the ways in which children and young people could be better supported in their education and social care.

Further reading

Alexandre-Passe, N (2015a) *Dyslexia and Mental Health*. London: Jessica Kingsley Publications.

This book is unusual in its approach to dyslexia. Alexander-Passe is an experienced researcher in dyslexia, but as a teacher of special needs children, and someone who is dyslexic himself, he has approached the subject with first-hand knowledge of what it feels like to be dyslexic and offers a discussion of the intervention strategies that really work. The book sensitively approaches many real-life examples of the physical and mental health challenges that someone identified with dyslexia may encounter when living in a non-dyslexic world.

The book asks the reader to consider whether dyslexia is a social/psychological issue (manifested by a reading society), or a combination of neurological deficits, in other words whether this is 'nature or nurture'. Alexander-Passe encourages all those who are dyslexic to talk freely about their experiences to start their own 'healing' process.

References

Alexandre-Passe, N (2015a) *Dyslexia and Mental Health*. London: Jessica Kingsley Publications.

Alexandre-Passe, N (2015b) Dyslexia: investigating self-harm and suicidal thoughts/ attempts as a coping strategy. *Journal of Psychology and Psychotherapy*. https://www.researchgate.net/publication/290213848_Dyslexia_Investigating_Self-Harm_and_Suicidal_ThoughtsAttempts_as_a_Coping_Strategy (accessed 24. 11. 19).

Boyes, M, Leitao, S, Claessen, M, Badcock, A and Noyton, M (2016) Why are reading difficulties associated with mental health problems? *Dyslexia* 22: 263–266.

Dahle, AE and Knivsberg, A (2015) *Internalizing and Externalizing Attention Problems in Dyslexia*. National Center for Reading and Educational Research. Norway: University of Stavanger. www.researchgate.net/publication/271755320_Internalizing_externalizing_and_attention_problems_in_dyslexia (accessed 20. 11. 19).

Easton, P, Entwhistle, V and Williams, B (2013) How the stigma of low literacy can impair patient – professional spoken interactions and affect health: insights from a qualitative investigation. *BMC Health Services Research* 13: 319https://bmchealthservres.biomedcentral.com/articles/10.1186/1472-6963-13-319 (accessed 30. 11. 19).

Edwards, J (1994) *The Scars of Dyslexia*. London: Cassell.

Elmer, N (2001) *The Costs and Causes of Low Self Esteem*. York: Rowntree.

Hampshire, S (1990) *Every Letter Counts*. London: Corgi.

Hawton, K, Rodham, K, Evans, E and Weatherall, R (2002) Deliberate self harm in adolescents: self report survey in school in England. *British Medical Journal* 325: 1207–1211.

Henderson, DA and Thompson, CL (2016) *Counselling Children* (9th edn). Boston: Cengage Learning.

Knapp, M, McDaid, D and Parsonage, M (eds) (2011) *Mental Health Promotion and Mental Illness Prevention: The Economic Case*. PSSRU. London: London School of Economics and Political Science; Department of Health.

Mind (2013) *Mental Health Facts and Statistics*. www.mind.org.uk (accessed 21. 11. 19).

Morris, D and Turnball, P (2006) Clinical experiences of students with dyslexia. *Radiography* 15(4): 341–344.

National Audit Office (2014) *Children in Care*. London: NAO Communications.

National Health Service (2019) *Clinical Depression*. www.nhs.uk (accessed 22. 11. 19).

National Institute for Health and Care Excellence (NICE) (2015) *Costing Statement (NG27)*. www.nice.org.uk/guidance/ng27/resources/costing-statement-2187244909 (accessed 30. 11. 19).

Newlands F, Shrewsbury D and Robson J (2014) Foundation doctors and dyslexia: a qualitative study of their experiences and coping strategies. *Postgraduate Medical Journal* 91: 121–126.

Office for National Statistics (2018) *Suicides in UK: 2017 Registrations*. www.ons.gov.uk/peoplepopulationandcommunity/healthandsocialcare (accessed 30. 11. 19).

Palmer, S, Dainow, S and Milner, P (eds) (1996) *The BAC Counselling Reader*. London: Sage.

Reid, G (2017) *Dyslexia in the Early Years: A Handbook for Practice*. London: Jessica Kingsley Publications.

Riddick, B (2010) *Living with Dyslexia* (2nd edn). Abingdon: Routledge.

Scott, R (2004) *Dyslexia and Counselling*. London: Whurr Publications.

Shaw, SCK and Anderson, JL (2017) The experiences of medical students with dyslexia: an interpretive phenomenological study. *Dyslexia* 24: 220–233.

Shaywitz, S (2005) *Overcoming Dyslexia*. New York: Vintage Books.

Thomson, M (1996) *Developmental Dyslexia: Studies in Disorders of Communication*. London: Whurr Publications.

Tsiachristas, A, McDaid, D, Casey, D, Brand, F, Leal, J, Parl, A-La, Geulayov, G and Hawton, K (2017) General hospital costs in England of medical and psychiatric care for patients who self-harm: a retrospective analysis. *The Lancet Psychiatry* 4. www.thelancet.com/psychiatry (accessed 21. 11. 19).

Willcutt, E and Gaffney-Brown, R (2004) Etiology of dyslexia, ADHD and related difficulties. *Perspectives* 30: 12–15.

5 The cost to education and social service

Introduction

Education has always been accepted as one of the ways to use the national wealth to provide opportunities for all. It has over the years been seen by all party-political persuasions as a tool of reform, as a social leveller and a way of providing equality of opportunity. However, this can only be achieved if those working within the system have sufficient training and awareness of the implications of IPDs and how influential they can be to future lives. Contrary to much public thinking, sending a child to school in the UK is not compulsory and home schooling is perfectly legal in the UK; the requirement is that every child, including those with special needs, receives a full-time education. It is therefore crucial for those who are within the school system that we get it 'right' and fit for purpose for each unique individual.

> When we make laws which compel our children to go to school, we assume collectively an awesome responsibility. For a period of some ten years, the children are conscripts.
>
> (Donaldson, 1978, p. 13)

This chapter will focus on the need to train teachers, practitioners and those working in social services. It will draw upon small-scale research undertaken in 2017 (Hayes, 2018) concerning the limited awareness and training of teachers and practitioners working in early years. This will be set against the need to produce sensitive and knowledgeable teachers and social workers who understand the process of learning and the wide-ranging impact that information processing differences (IPDs) can have upon this.

Policy implementation

During the many interviews conducted for the research for this book, and despite the many and inclusive definitions of dyslexia, it is clear that the biggest challenges for the individual with dyslexia lie in their school days. It is their school years that most of the interviewees wanted to talk about, this was the time when the focus of their dyslexia was most heightened. The school years were the ones which either enable them to have the resilience to overcome the challenges which they carried forward with them to adulthood or was the time when they lost all confidence in themselves and their ability to achieve at any level. For this reason, schools and those who work in them, teachers, practitioners and teaching assistants, carry a very heavy burden of responsibility. What happens in schools and nurseries is likely to live with a person for the rest of their lives; it shapes their careers, relationships and expectations. This makes it all the more surprising that teachers, practitioners and teaching assistants have a very limited understanding of IPDs and, importantly, how to approach any sort of intervention programme. In 2017 I conducted a piece of small-scale research of a random sample of teachers, practitioners and teaching assistants, which clearly indicated the level of confusion that exists within these professions of what dyslexia really is. When asked to define the condition almost all believed that it was to do with reading and literacy, but most did not understand that it was a holistic condition relating to a far wider range of manifestations than just reading (Hayes, 2018).

Reid (2016) stresses the importance of local education authorities developing a coherent and agreed definition upon which to base all their provision, and upon which their teachers and practitioners can develop their practice and intervention techniques. Each local education authority needs to have a clearly defined policy for working with children with IPDs, which needs to take account of a number of issues. According to Reid (2016), each policy should have:

1   A clear and consistently recognisable definition of dyslexia and IPDs, which is agreed throughout their documentation.
2   A coherent way to identify children at risk, and recognise the wide variations that exist on this spectrum of learning differences.
3   A means to recognise that different areas of the curriculum are likely to impact upon children in different ways, both positively and negatively.
4   A means to recognise the importance of parents and families, both to the initial identification and later ongoing support.
5   The ability to recognise the holistic nature of the impact upon the children, and how any intervention and support needs to take account of the all-round development of the child.
6   The means to recognise the imperative for continuing professional development for *all* staff, including non-teaching staff, who are supporting children with IPDs.
7   The means to support the development of intervention programmes, that have been shown to work for the needs of each unique child as an individual, at differing stages of their development and school career.
8   At *least* one specially trained and experienced member of staff in every setting, to lead the identification and support, and to act as a portal of knowledge for those in the setting to draw upon, confide in and consult with.

9   A balance of provision of resources and support strategies in mainstream provision (with specialist staff) and specialist units.
10 Details of strategies and training to ensure the approachability of staff in all settings.
11 Responsive assessment and formal identification processes suited to the needs of the child.

In the research by Hayes (2018), it was clear that most teachers and childcare practitioners did not believe that they had sufficient teaching in their initial training programmes to fully understand how to support children with IPDs, and the methodology and strategies that could be used to help their pupils. In a search of the relevant literature, Reid (2016) found that in some instances even the university lecturers, who were teaching teachers, knew less about dyslexia than their students! He also found that there were wild inconsistencies between one teacher training institution and another, even in the definition of dyslexia and the intervention strategies that they considered work best. Considering the widespread prevalence of IPDs in schools and colleges, this is only likely to produce confusion amongst frontline staff, and consternation about their preparedness to deal with the challenges in an appropriate manner.

REFLECT ON THIS

1   List the barriers that you believe exist, which would prevent such a policy from being developed consistently by local education authorities.
2   List the barriers that you believe exist, which would prevent the consistent implementation of such a policy by frontline staff. Consider each point in turn and discuss with a colleague.
3   How far do you believe that financial restraints will restrict the implementation of each item on the list?

Identification

Adults with dyslexia frequently cite, as a major issue, the education personnel who failed to identify their learning differences whilst in school. A very common scenario is the grandparent who watches their grandchildren struggling in school, the grandchild may be undergoing assessment and is eventually identified as dyslexic. The adult relates this to their own life and realises that their own struggles in school were probably caused by a lack of recognition of their own dyslexia in their youth, and for some they become very resentful of the pain and distress that this has caused. It would be fine to think that this lack of identification was a thing of the past, but I know that with each intake of higher education students to university, there will be a proportion who have not been identified during their school career. Upon submitting their first assignment it is clear that they have struggled with their written communication, and upon assessment at the age of eighteen or above, they are identified, and appropriate support put in place to allow them to compete on equal terms with their non-dyslexic colleagues and peers. Hayes (2018) argues that if this, as is likely, is a genetic condition then we are born with it and die with it, so if practitioners and childcarers working in early years had the knowledge themselves, it is possible that many children could be identified as at risk of an IPD at a very early stage in their development, certainly long before children are starting to fail to read. It should be noted that at such an early age this identification would not be a diagnosis or labelling of dyslexia or any other IPD, but a consideration of the level of risk that a particular child may have of going on to develop an IPD. This could be done through observation, listening to the child's families, and a knowledge-based understanding rather than formal testing and assessment. This method of observational assessment does not rely upon a deficit model of dyslexia, it does not require professionals to wait until it is clear that a child cannot do something before intervention, but rather looks at the whole child, at both positive and negative indications of an IPD. There is always going to be a risk of false positives and false negatives, in what some experts would regard as a rather 'woolly' and over-inclusive means of identification, but as this is likely to be an ongoing observational assessment, gradually these will filter out, and the children in most need of intervention strategies will have been supported long before their sense of failure and low self-esteem can have started to impact upon their lives, and more formal and traditional assessments from a specialist teacher or educational psychologists can then be employed.

Inclusion

In the last ten to fifteen years the emphasis of policy for special educational need (SEN) has been upon inclusion and integration of children with particular needs into a mainstream classroom. Children with an ever-widening range of special needs are taught alongside mainstream children by teachers and practitioners with no, or limited, training or understanding of the resource needs of the full range of disorders, disabilities and differences that their children present with. Certainly, integrating all children within a classroom promotes a positive message about diversity and tolerance within society, but it is important to constantly question the ability of generalist teachers and practitioners, some of whom will be young and inexperienced, to achieve every child's maximum potential and it is questionable whether it is even fair or reasonable to expect teachers and practitioners to be all things to all children. This is especially so when a constantly narrowing curriculum is being demanded by the government, with a continual emphasis upon raising standards within a small number of subject areas, which may not suit, or even be appropriate for all children, particularly those with special educational needs (SEND).

In 2000 the Qualifications and Curriculum Authority (QCA) put forward three key principles for inclusion:

- Setting suitable learning challenges
- Responding to students' diverse learning needs
- Overcoming potential barriers to learning and assessment for individuals and groups of students.

However, for children with dyslexia the whole concept of inclusion is such a movable feast, and can mean so many different things, from the child with an IPD in a mainstream classroom supported by a mainstream teacher with no specialist knowledge, to a discrete setting were all the children are similarly assessed and identified with specialist teachers for a particular condition. There is also a great deal of middle ground, and variations on these, for example, separate units sited within a school, children in mainstream withdrawn for periods of the day for specialist support, and children in mainstream withdrawn for periods of time with non-specialist support etc. However, one could argue, using the QCA principles, that neither of these assumptions is really fully inclusive, but rather exclusive and selective, taking the children away from their peers and mainstream experiences.

Since the 1988 Education Act, all children taught in every state funded school in England are required to learn a similar set of detailed subject related skills, knowledge and understanding. The National Curriculum lays down a statutory entitlement for all children to be taught to these standards and only in exceptional circumstances can a child be excused from all or part of the National Curriculum.

Although the National Curriculum provides a minimum for what must be taught, it does not state *how* it might be taught, although guidance is available, it is just that, guidance, and it is for individual schools and individual teachers to choose how they organise their teaching programmes. Such a rigidly proposed curriculum can, however, present difficulties for a teacher faced with thirty-five children in a class, all unique and individual, all beginning from a different starting point, with different experiences, different expectations of education, different cultures, varying levels of parental interest, varying intellectual levels and different ways of processing the information they receive from that environment. Although the numbers of children with dyslexia and IPDs are not calculated exactly, and its prevalence is highly contested even by the experts, it is generally agreed that the likelihood is that every school, and probably every classroom, will have children with IPDs in them, it is therefore critical that those working with them understand how best to meet their needs, socially, emotionally, physically and cognitively.

Before the 1980s it was likely that every child identified with a learning difficulty would be educated in a specialist school. However, since then there has been a growing awareness of the need to widen access to mainstream schooling, and there is now an expectation that most children will be integrated into mainstream settings. A child formally assessed as dyslexic should be registered on a school's special educational needs register and the school must respond within the framework of the Special Educational Needs Code of

Practice (DfE/DoH: 2015). The special educational needs coordinator (SENCO) will coordinate the advice given by professionals with a close partnership with parents and carers. The SENCO is then responsible for overseeing the child's needs, to ensure that appropriate resources and provision are in place. An Education and Health Care Plan will then be drawn up with clear and measurable targets, to ensure that all staff are aware of the needs of the child and there is a requirement that these should be reviewed regularly, usually termly.

Some schools staff and parents have expressed serious concerns about inclusion being right for all children, including the majority of the children in the class who could be disrupted by a child with difficult to manage behaviour, or not receive the full attention of a teacher or a teaching assistant who will be diverted to support the child with the particular needs. There could be concerns about a blanket, uncompromising policy, which could divert financial resources from the mainstream children to support the child with additional needs. There are certainly concerns from staff and parents that the mainstream schools do not have the facilities, skills, knowledge and understanding of conditions to really be able to support children in mainstream. Time is always an issue for teachers, when they have a class of thirty-five children; they may feel that they do not have sufficient time to devote to one child who constantly struggles with the pace and the rigors of learning to read for example. I am certainly not arguing for children with IPDs to be segregated and put into discrete specialist settings, although for some children this is certainly beneficial and specialist schools such as the Red Rose School in Lancashire, work hard with children who have failed to thrive in a mainstream setting. This particular specialist school was co-founded by Gavin Reid, a psychologist and leading authority in this area of special education, and all staff working there are trained and experienced in IPDs. Schools such as the Red Rose are independent of the state sector and as such are a very expensive option and probably not open to many families. There are some non-fee-paying schools which specialise in this area, but there are not many, and a more likely option would be a mainstream school with a British Dyslexia Association Dyslexia Friendly Quality Mark, or a school registered with the Council for the Registration of Schools Teaching Dyslexic Pupils (CReSTeD); this recognises that a school has dyslexia friendly practice in place, with all staff aware of the particular needs of those with dyslexia and able to support appropriately. It was in 2001 when Neil Mackay coined the phrase Dyslexia Friendly; he wrote about his experiences in a secondary school in North Wales, where he had considerable success working with children with dyslexia at GCSE level (Mackay, 2012). This was picked up by the British Dyslexia Association (BDA), and they developed an authority-wide Dyslexia Friendly Plan, which has since become associated with a mark of quality for those schools and organisations that offer a framework of support and understanding for children and adults with dyslexia.

However, inclusion is controversial and educational settings do need to question their ability to ensure that they can adequately provide for the needs of a child, and ensure that neither the physical environment of the setting nor the behaviour and understanding of the staff can lead to a child being even further disadvantaged by their condition. There is no easy answer to an issue which presents moral and ethical questions, which need to be under constant review. It is likely that extremely disruptive children with unpredictable reactions, disorganisation and acute impulsivity, such as might be seen with ADD or ADHD, are unlikely to be taught effectively in mainstream classrooms without adversely impacting the education of the other children. The disproportionate levels of time, ingenuity and effort required for such children could detract from what the staff can give to the majority of children in the class. Interestingly the Centre for Studies in Inclusive Education (CSIE, 1995) does not take such a pragmatic approach:

> Regular schools with this inclusive orientation are the most effective means of combating discriminatory attitudes, creating welcoming communities, building on an inclusive society and achieving education for all; moreover, they provide an effective education to the majority of children and improve the efficiency and ultimately the cost effectiveness of the entire education system.
> (CSIE, 1995, p. 80)

Teachers and practitioners generally embrace the concept of inclusion, but in discussion with some it is also clear that they are concerned about the levels of support and resources that they are able to offer; many also have concerns about their own levels of training and whether they had sufficient skills to ensure that the children in their care have the best support. General teaching programmes such as the Post Graduate Certificate in Education (PGCE) do not usually have the time, or even tutor expertise, to ensure that trainees have the understanding of special education that they really need, and in-service training is expensive and totally reliant upon teachers' special interests and willingness to engage; this is often in their own time and at their own expense.

Avramidis and Norwich (2002) showed that teachers' attitudes depended upon three intersecting themes (Figure 5.1):

1   *Child related variables*: how severe is the nature of the learning differences, their behaviour and physical capabilities, and how much it impacts upon their time and the progress of the other children.
2   *Teacher related variables*: such as an interest in the subject area and willingness to work with children with special needs.
3   *Context/environment*: are the appropriate resources available, provided by the local education authorities and employers, such as, additional staff, suitable equipment and the overall willingness of other staff in the setting.

In the current system, once a special educational need is formally identified in a child, the local authority is obliged to take some action, and this is likely to be expensive on resources, both human and physical. However, it is possible that this

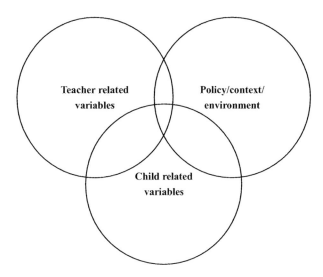

Figure 5.1 Variables to inclusive practice
Adapted from Avramidis and Norwich (2002)

could also be working in a negative manner for children with an IPD, as local authorities delay or even deny the very existence of the special need, often for financial reasons. An example of this has recently been reported in the national press that dyslexia is no longer to be identified by some local authorities (Bodkin, 2019). Warwickshire and Staffordshire claimed, in 2019, that the science behind dyslexia was questionable, and therefore they would not be making assessments available in schools, to the children in their care, they have since been encouraged to review this policy (Bodkin, 2019). They do not believe that it is important to distinguish between children with dyslexia and those who have more generalised learning difficulties and are struggling to read. This sort of action by local authorities results in individual parents taking action and even instigating expensive tribunals to fight what they see as unfair decisions and even discrimination. These tribunals are often very frightening for the lay person, David and Goliath battles, which are often highly technical, legalistic and weighted against a parent with no knowledge of such quasi-legal proceedings. Scott (2004) suggests that local authorities rely on the fact that only a very small minority of parents will attempt to go this far. It is likely, though not exclusively so, that those who do will be professional, well-educated, middle classers, who have an above average income to employ legal representation to support their complaints.

> For the few who take on the stress involved in appealing, a hundred of these will fall by the wayside, unable to cope with the time, potential expense and mind-numbing complexities of dealing with council lawyers.
> (Scott, 2004, p. 2004)

Inclusion may indeed work for some children some of the time, but it is unlikely to work for all the children all the time.

REFLECT ON THIS

1 Work with a colleague to write down what inclusion means to you.
2 Compare this to the inclusion policy in your setting, or one known to you. How is this understanding of inclusion similar to yours, or does it differ?

Abuse

As shocking as it may seem, many children with an IPD report that they experienced emotional, verbal and even physical abuse in school from teachers. Scott (2004) suggests that all children with dyslexia experienced some form of damage, just by going to school. She describes school for some children as *torture*, both psychologically and physically, which is a very strong sentiment. She also believes that a child's experience of school can be humiliating and degrading, with children having to cope with the *raw brutality* of such very public failure. She suggests that collectively as a society we should be ashamed.

Perhaps teachers prefer *easy children,* ones who are no trouble to them, as they believe that this affirms their success as a teacher. The very word 'teacher' implies learning, after all we cannot be said to have taught something unless someone has learned. Working with teachers, teaching assistants and practitioners for many years, I frequently heard them say *I have been teaching him all week and he still doesn't seem to understand!* This is clearly an oxymoron, because if they had taught something then clearly the child would have learned, and if they have not learned, they have not been taught.

Interview

Leon is now in his thirties and has had a successful career in the army. He recalls incidents from his traumatic primary school days.

> I was only seven years old and in a small rural primary school. The teacher was always on at me to 'catch up', 'pay attention' and 'work harder'. I tried, I really, really tried, but the harder I tried the harder it seemed to be to read the words on the page. I was always at the back of the class and I don't remember the teacher ever saying anything nice to or about me. It was always that I was stupid and lazy. The teacher was a man, probably in his forties, and he would come up to me and pull back my head by grabbing my hair. He would shout right on my face, and I could feel his spit on my face. I can remember it now as clear as day. He would go so red in the face. As I look back I realise that he was probably frustrated with me and couldn't think why his teaching was not getting through to me. One day he got so cross he threw a ruler at me and caught me on the arm.

We had a big green 'blackboard' on an easel, one day he got so cross with me that he swept it aside and the whole thing landed on a desk and broke the desk. That broken desk stayed at the back of the classroom for as long as I was in the school and was always a reminder to me, each day, of how frightened I was of him.

When I look back, I realise that this was really wrong and was abuse, but when you are only seven years old you don't think like that. He was an adult and a teacher; I couldn't even tell my mum as I was too afraid that I would get into trouble because after all, it was all my fault ... or that is how it felt!

On 8 July 2011 The Daily Mail newspaper reported (Lawson, 2011) that a school boy, Lawrence Manning, took his own life after being pushed and poked in the chest by a teacher; the coroner's court considered that he was suffering from post-traumatic stress due to the abuse by the teacher, and that the abuse of the power differential resulted in both humiliation and fear. Edwards (1994) records a number of other cases of negative feelings and violence from teachers to children with dyslexia, for example, John who recounts being hit with a broom, and Trevor who believes that he was regularly insulted and humiliated by staff in his school. George (Edwards, 1994) claims that he was pushed into a corner so violently by the teacher that he banged his head and Oliver was put in a corner and forgotten about. It is small wonder that Scott (2004) believes that many children with IPDs go on to develop school phobia as a form of coping strategy, either refusing to attend school or truanting.

Classrooms are, at the same time, both very public and very private places, and teachers conduct in a classroom is seen by twenty to forty children and young people every day, but rarely by another adult, so the teacher is seldom held accountable for their actions, as the children often regard the behaviour as either *normal* for teachers, and must be endured, or that no one will believe them anyway. This makes it very difficult for children and their parents to seek any redress for the teacher's abusive behaviour particularly with very young children. Children are generally very trusting beings and want to try to 'fit in', so they do not complain. The sort of abuse described above by the interviewee is such that would be completely unacceptable and unlawful in any other walk of life, and means that for some children school is not a safe place to be, causing stress and in some cases psychopathology (Scott, 2004).

> What is clear is that most dyslexics spend their time at school veering between fear and outright terror it is hardly surprising that they fail to thrive.
> (Scott, 2004, p. 55)

Unfortunately, it is probably true that, without appropriate quality support, many children with dyslexia, and their very different levels of brain organisation, are likely to fail everything that our education holds dear, as almost everything relies upon being able to read well, to write, spell, organise themselves, listen to instruction and take responsibility for their possessions.

Assessment

A report by Dyslexia Action (2012) showed that according to the parents interviewed, 61% of children had to wait for a year or more for support following their dyslexia identification, and 90% of the parents surveyed believed that the teachers lacked the necessary awareness of the condition. Following the report Dyslexia Awareness called for all teachers to have appropriate teaching during their initial training, to support the children most at risk; they suggest that as these conditions are so prevalent there should be, at least, a compulsory module on dyslexia and special educational needs.

> We undertook this exercise to assess how much progress had been made over the last 40 years. Despite the improved understanding of dyslexia and the techniques that work, we were shocked to learn that so many parents reported that their schools are still unwilling to recognise dyslexia and take action to support dyslexic children. While the government may recognise dyslexia as a genuine condition, and if unaddressed, as a significant contributor to poor academic progress, it is a tragedy that this knowledge is not more widely shared amongst individual school teachers.
> (Dyslexia Action, 2012, p. 56)

> It is less costly, to both the individual and society, to provide appropriate help at the earliest possible time. The current cost to the economy of under employment, unemployment and crime, is billions of pounds every year.
> (Dyslexia Action, 2012, p. 56)

The parents who took part in the Dyslexia Action (2012) survey highlighted a particular issue in the transition between Key Stage Two and Key Stage Three, the point at which most children transition from primary to secondary education. They believed that what was needed was a whole school community approach to assist with the trauma of that transition, including appropriate training for teaching assistants, mid-day supervisors and before- and after-school club supervisors, to enable them to support a much larger percentage of the children in a more holistic manner throughout the school day. Research by the Driver Youth Trust (2015) showed that up to a third of local authorities reported a shortfall in the number of teachers with specialist dyslexia skills, knowledge and understanding. In 2009, the government of the day pledged £10 million to train these teachers, but the research suggests that ten years later, only half of that money was spent (Driver Youth Trust, 2015). This same report showed that finance and support varies widely between local authorities, making it very much a postcode lottery for those who believe that they are entitled to access that support.

It is clear from talking to people who either have, or have close connections to, dyslexia, that despite the very centralized system of education in England, with the National Curriculum and nationally organised Standard Assessment Tasks (SATS), that their experiences of the system vary widely. There are huge variations between three different areas of that system:

1   Local authority policy making
2   Schools
3   Individual teachers.

This variation means that individuals often get very different experiences of educational quality depending upon where in the country they live, which schools they either elect to attend or are allocated and even which year teachers they are taught by.

Education, Health and Care plans

An Education, Health and Care (EHC) plan is a legally enforceable document that stipulates the health, education and care needs of a child with special educational needs, and the support they should receive to fulfil their potential. Following an EHC assessment, this will be drawn up and reviewed annually by the local authority. According to the Department for Education (2018), there is an increasing number of children with special educational needs. There are currently 1.3 million children in England with special educational needs, which is approximately 14% of the whole school population. However, only about 253,680 have either a special educational needs statement or an EHC plan, and over 28% of these have autistic spectrum disorders. A further 1,022,535 children are on special educational needs support. So many do not have their particular needs recognised formally by the school, and many are excluded, or home schooled, whilst waiting for suitable assessment and provision; on occasions, this may take years. The charity Ambitious about Autism, in their impact report of 2013–2014, claim that some children with special educational needs are being removed from school rolls either temporarily, on fixed term exclusions, or permanently, due to the financial pressures within the school, or to improve the appearance of their academic success (Ambitious about Autism, 2014). This is a process often referred to as *off-rolling* and is especially apparent when behavioural issues threaten inspection results. Timpson (2019) heavily criticized the practice of off-rolling, describing it as *simply wrong*; however, he believed that if it was stopped it could result in a rise in formal exclusions, and possibly even deter some schools from admitting children with conditions that could result in poor behaviour, even though that practice, if proven, could be illegal. Timpson describes off-rolling as:

> The practice of removing a pupil from the school roll without a formal, permanent exclusion or by encouraging a parent to remove their child from the school roll, when the removal is primarily in the interests of the school rather than in the best interests of the pupil. Off-rolling in these circumstances is a form of 'gaming'.
>
> (Timpson 2019, p. 100)

Timpson (2019) also found evidence that pressure was being put upon some parents to move their child to another school, what was seen as a 'managed move', which merely shunted the difficulty into another system, without tackling the underlying difficulties. According to the Timpson Review for the Department for Education (Timpson, 2019), 46.7% of children with special educational needs were permanently excluded in 2016–2017, this is six times higher than non-SEND children. The impact of this upon families and employment is huge, with up to 30% of families reporting that one or more of them either gave up work to care for their SEND children or went part-time. Almost a third of these families admitted that they had missed days from work in the last year. This same report showed that exclusions for children on the autistic spectrum had increased by nearly 60% since 2011.

Funding

In July 2018 the Education and Skills Funding Agency produced a National Funding formula (NFF), which meant that funding for schools is now based on *individual need and characteristics of every school in the country* (Education and Skills Funding Agency, 2018, p. 3). This means that whilst there is a basic per-pupil entitlement to funding, depending upon age and Key Stage, there is additional funding, within each state funded school, for every SEND child in their care. However, in the UK academic expectations are undoubtably linked to education expenditure and although teachers are a deserving and admirable group of people, relatively they are not highly paid, but despite searching the literature, there appears to be very little evidence that increasing school finances significantly improves a child's chances of learning to read. For the financial year 2019–2020 the predicted total education budget in the UK was £87.2 billion, which is a considerable proportion of tax payers' finance, and understandably the public want to see accountability and value for money.

REFLECT ON THIS

The importance of school and education to a child cannot be emphasised enough, and it has the potential to influence a child for the rest of their life, both positively and negatively. Scott (2004) makes some very profound judgements about schools in this country, including the following statement:

> When life goes wrong for a child in school, their life goes wrong for a long time after they leave school. The influence of school is profound.
> (Scott, 2004, p. 53).

1 How far do you agree with this statement from Scott (2004)?
2 In your opinion is such a profound influence ever irreversible?

3   Reflect on your own experiences in school or education; how do you believe it impacted your life long after you left?
4   Draw up a table of both positive and negative experiences that you had in school which resulted in long term changes to you and your behaviour.

Social services

It is incumbent on every school to provide an inclusive environment where every child feels welcomed and respected, enabling them to achieve their potential, and this is likely to mean a multiagency approach to inclusion. Traditionally schools are concerned with education and social services are concerned with a child's home background and parental circumstances, and neither agency invades the other's space. In an ideal world these two agencies (and others) should be working closely together to provide a holistic support experience for the child; however, whilst today there is usually some contact between social services and education, it is clear in a number of high-profile cases, some recorded in the Munro Review (2011), that this multiagency communication is not always as effective as necessary, to prevent children from slipping between the agencies.

It is highly likely that social workers will regularly come into contact with service users who have a range of IPDs, so understanding how a condition such as dyslexia can impact the lives of the service user, and their family dynamics holistically, is really vital to the quality of any relationship that they may be able to build between them. Social workers need to be aware of the key role that they can play in helping their service user manage their dyslexia, and the challenges that often come with that; they need to understand that this is *not* just an educational problem for teachers to address, but could potentially be at the heart of so many of the challenges that their service user has faced throughout their life. Social workers will often have to work with people with mental health problems, severe anxiety, depression and psychotic illnesses, which can result in them displaying challenging behaviours, but are often not looking behind the behaviour to the source of the difficulties. They need to understand that dyslexia and IPDs are often hidden disabilities, with adults either not knowing that they have an IPD or are deliberately concealing for fear of admitting to what they see as a stigmatised identity. One aspect of the work of social services is to provide a voice for the vulnerable, ridiculed and victimized, and it is often mental illness that brings people to the attention of social services.

According to the Association of Directors of Adult Social Services (ADASS) (2019), there are ever increasing pressures on frontline social services and social workers to have the understanding, knowledge and skills to meet the needs of vulnerable families with an ever dwindling financial pot. However, for most social workers in their initial training, there is little guidance or even awareness raising of families and individuals with low literacy and IPDs. Some social workers may receive continuing professional development (CPD) and training in this field but others report that they feel that there is a lack of relevant training available. A small, hitherto unpublished survey (thirty-four participants), which I conducted with my social work students in 2018 (Figure 5.2), clearly indicated that they felt very unprepared for working with and recognising issues of dyslexia and low literacy. The survey indicated that most were unaware of how dyslexia and IPDs could impact their service users in such a holistic manner, believing that dyslexia was an issue for education concerned with reading.

Research by Nalavany et al. (2015) showed that there was almost no research focused on dyslexia for social workers, despite the fact that dyslexia clearly *fits within the social work mandate* (Nalavany et al., 2015, p. 568).

> A competent social worker who understands the depth of pain from early and present experiences of the adult with dyslexia may play a role in the lives of these individuals that is every bit as important as the role of the competent educator.
>
> (Nalavany et al., 2015, p. 569)

If a social worker suspects that the service user that they are working with is dyslexic, or has low literacy, probably one of the most useful things that they can do is to support them to arrange an assessment, and by identifying their difficulties they can help to boost their self-esteem, which is often a gateway to the rest of their lives when they can say: *Oh … now I understand why I was like that in school*. Initially, such an assessment is going to be expensive (probably £400–£600 per service user), but could make a huge change in that person's life and possibly allow them to understand their difficulties in a very different way, which could lead to them receiving training, returning to employment, improving mental health, etc. Assessments can sometimes be arranged through a GP, if they believe that it is negatively impacting the heath of their patient, so close ties with the health service may be useful. Munro (2011) recognised in

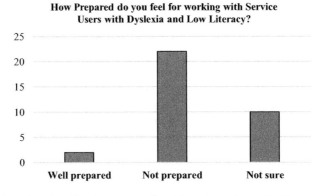

Figure 5.2 Results of small-scale survey of social work students (2018)

her review that financial pressures were placing interagency training in jeopardy, and she called for more funding for multi-agency training, as she witnessed an increasing polarisation of education, health and social services. She recognised that such separation could only be detrimental to the support offered to children.

The local job centre can also sometimes make a referral for an assessment, or if someone is already employed they can be helped to have frank discussions with their employer, or their human resources department. Students can be encouraged to find help through their college or university departments for inclusion and diversity. However, the social worker must never underestimate the worries about disclosure that some people may have, particularly if this *secret* has been kept from family, friends and employers for a very long time.

It is unlikely that a service user who is dyslexic will disclose this to the social worker in the initial stages of their relationship, not at least without some prompting, even for those who *are* aware of their dyslexia and suspect that this is the source of many of the difficulties and problems that they face. Without knowledge of a service user's IPD the social worker is really working in the dark, as so much important information is lost by not establishing this one fact from the outset of the relationship. It is vital that the social worker understands the life pathway which has led this service user to come to the attention of the authorities. Communication is probably at the heart of what a social worker does, but if the service user is unable to understand what their supporter is talking about, cannot read the information, cannot organise their thoughts or sequence what they are being told, then that communication and that relationship breaks down. The service user who has any sort of IPD needs a time lag built into their communication string, to be able to fully understand, and a creative and insightful supporter to be innovative with their methods of communication. The social worker may need to speak more slowly and clearly, use concrete examples such as illustrations, spider grams, diagrams and pictures, and be empathetic to the problems that differences of short-term memory retention can make to understanding and ability to organise their life. With the average salary of a trained and experienced social worker in 2019 ranging from £28,370 to £46,462, they are not particularly well paid for the immense responsibilities that society asks them to shoulder.

Figure 5.3 shows the results of a survey conducted with my social work students in 2018. This is a possible indicator of their limited understanding of the multifarious nature of dyslexia and the holistic impact that this could potentially have on their service users.

Case study

Anja is an experienced social worker. She and her son have been assessed by the BDA as being dyslexic, but she was a gifted student and found ways to get around her difficulties. Like many other children she struggled with written work, but had high powers of recall and excellent verbal skills, which she used very ably from

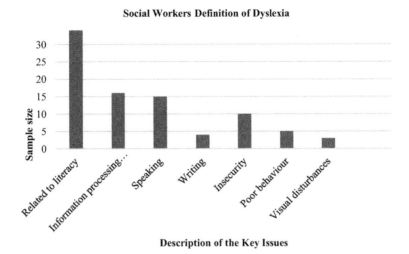

Figure 5.3 Small-scale survey of thirty-four social work students' understanding of dyslexia

childhood, for example by talking her way out of having to write. She struggled with her social work training but had a lot of support from the university that she attended. She claims to have had no training in dealing with service users who have IPDs but feels that she has an empathy with them. She has had a variety of experiences in social care settings with children and young people who she now thinks could have also been struggling with their literacy.

She had many negative feelings about her days in education and developed an involvement with her local community using photography to aid communication. She had a few difficulties within her training placements because of her verbal, reflective and analytical skills. Her assessments were all passes, but she required longer to write any assignment, report or social work duty/intake referral notes. Her spelling is poor, and she lacks confidence in her abilities. Levels of organisation are difficult, with time keeping and appointments, and this caused her further anxiety and word muddle.

Chapter reflections

To view dyslexia and other IPDs only as an educational issue is certainly shortsighted; it fails to recognise these as lifelong conditions which can pervade the whole person. Schooling and education, whilst an extremely important and potentially formative time of a child's life, form only a relatively short period in the life of an individual, although this is a time when these conditions are probably most significant and have the potential to do the most harm to an individual's mental health and future personality. However, support beyond childhood can often play a crucial role in enhancing an individual's self-esteem and overall feeling of well-being.

To ensure adequate provision for an individual with an IPD is likely to involve a multidisciplinary approach, with people who know how to support them and make reasonable adjustments to enable that support, often diverting people to other agencies such as health, education, social care services, employer's groups, charitable institutions and voluntary groups. Social workers and teachers need to be trained and ready to meet a full range of complex and diverse needs in those that they care for, and considering the likely prevalence of dyslexia this needs to be on the curriculum of every social work degree and teacher training programme in the country.

The following chapter will look more closely at the high prevalence of dyslexia and low literacy within the criminal justice system and a pathway into criminality which so many find themselves when they have not developed that resilience and self-esteem.

Further reading

Nutbrown, C, Clough, P and Atherton, F (2013) *Inclusion in the Early Years*. London: Sage.

Although this book does focus upon children in the early years, it is an insightful and thought-provoking text, and the themes can be applied throughout the education system, which examines education within a political context. The book challenges long-held assumptions and practices of inclusion as an operational rather than conceptual process, and encourages the reader to question long-held and establishment ideas.

References

Ambitious About Autism (2014) *Making the Ordinary Possible*. www.ambitiousaboutautism.org.uk (accessed 01. 12. 19).

Association of Directors of Adult Social Services (ADASS) (2019) *ADASS Budget Survey 2019*. www.adass.org.uk/ (accessed 25. 11. 19).

Avramidis, E and Norwich, B (2002) Teachers' attitudes towards integration/inclusion: a review of literature. *European Journal of Special Needs Education* 17(2): 129–147.

Bodkin, H (2019) Dyslexia no longer being diagnosed by councils who called the disorder 'scientifically questionable'. *Daily Telegraph*, 11. 09. 19.

Centre for Studies in Inclusive Education (1995) *International Perspectives on Inclusion*. Bristol: CSIE.

Department for Education/Department of Health (2015) *Special Educational Needs and Disability Code of Practice 0 to 25: Statutory Guidance for Organisations which Work With and Support Children and Young People Who Have Special Educational Needs or Disabilities*. https://assets.publishing.service.gov.uk/government/uploads/system/uploads/attachment_data/file/398815/SEND_Code_of_Practice_January_2015.pdf (accessed 20.12.19.).

Department for Education (2018) *Special Educational Need in England: January 2018*. www.gov.uk/government/statistics/special-educational-needs-being-england-january-2018 (accessed 01. 12. 19).

Donaldson, M (1978) *Children's Mind*. London: Fontana.

Driver Youth Trust (2015) *Joining the Dots: Have Recent Reforms Worked For Those With SEND*. www.driveryouthtrust.com/wp-content/uploads/2018/07/DYT_JoinTheDotsReportOctober2015.pdf (accessed 29. 12. 19).

Dyslexia Action (2012) *Dyslexia Still Matters: Dyslexia in Our Schools Today, Progress Challenges and Solutions*. Surrey: Dyslexia Action.

Education and Skills Funding Agency (2018) *Schools Block Funding Formulae 2018–2019: Analysis of Local Authorities' Schools Block Funding Formulae*. London: Crown.

Edwards, J (1994) *The Scars of Dyslexia: Eight Case Studies in Emotional Reactions*. London: Cassell.

Hayes, C (2018) *Developmental Dyslexia from Birth to Eight Years: A Practitioner Guide*. Oxon: Routledge.

Lawson, P (2011) Dyslexic boy, 16, hanged himself after bullying by teachers at his primary school eight years earlier. *Daily Mail*, 08. 07. 11. www.dailymail.co.uk/news/article-2012654/Dyslexic-boy-16-hanged-bullying-teachers-primary-school-years-earlier.html (accessed 28. 11. 19).

Mackay, N (2012) *Removing Dyslexia as a Barrier to Achievement: The Dyslexia Friendly Schools Tool Kit*. Wakefield: SEN Marketing.

Munro, E (2011) *The Munro Review of Child Protection: Final report*. London: Department for Education.

Nalavany, BA, Carawan, LT and Sauber, S (2015) Adults with dyslexia, an invisible disability: the mediational role of concealment on perceived family support and self-esteem. *The British Journal of Social Work* 45(2): 568–586.

Nutbrown, C, Clough, P and Atherton, F (2013) *Inclusion in the Early Years*. London: Sage.

Qualifications and Curriculum Authority (QCA) (2000) *General Statement for Inclusion in Curriculum 2000*. London: QCA.

Reid, G (2016) *Dyslexia: A Practitioner's Handbook* (5th edn). Chichester: John Wiley and Sons.

Scott, R (2004) *Dyslexia and Counselling*. London: Whurr Publishers.

Timpson, E (2019) *Timpson Review of School Exclusion*. London: DfE.

6 The criminal justice system

Introduction

I am often asked by groups to talk about dyslexia and usually this involves the basic premises of what it might be, modern research and how prevalent it is. Almost always at the end people stay behind and want to ask questions that relate to themselves or their family. They frequently talk about the distress that they or a family member has experienced, and their 'battle' with authorities to get the condition recognised and appropriate quality support put in place. Many are very afraid of the direction in which a child might be taking, seeing the disaffection and negativity first-hand. They understand that this can, or already has, led to defiance, anti-social behaviour and even criminality. Frequently this can fracture relationships between parents and their children, especially as, from the child's perspective, their parents keep insisting upon sending them back to the school where they have been humiliated and bullied by teachers and peers alike. Saunders (1990) puts this succinctly when he says:

> Dyslexia won't kill you but it can mess up your life.
> (Saunders, 1990, p. 232)

This chapter will consider what is going on in our criminal justice system, and how prevalent low literacy and dyslexia are in our prisons and young offenders' institutions. The chapter will examine the links between dyslexia and criminality and the social and economic returns for providing appropriate, supportive, well-mentored environments where offenders can engage actively with literacy programmes, tailored to meet their particular needs.

Frustration, resentment and anger

When a young offender is initially identified with dyslexia their first reaction is often one of anger, that the education system that they struggled to engage with for so long could have let them down so badly (Kirk and Reid, 2003). They are angry with their school, their families and with society for not helping them to achieve; many young offenders have been moved from one

94 *The criminal justice system*

educational establishment to another, but have still not had their learning needs appropriately met. Alexander-Passe (2015) talks of young people with dyslexia in school watching their peers moving ahead of them: many of the peers will have high aspirations of higher education and eventually highly paid employment and social status, whilst those with dyslexia are often directed into a vocational career pathway, usually resulting in lower paid and less challenging employment. When they have lived under a cloud of believing that they are thick and stupid, it can be difficult to come to terms with how different things could have been.

> Schools tend to group low achieving students together, whether they have higher intelligence or not. They see low achievement and label accordingly. In addition, students who misbehave in class due to frustration or boredom are easily labelled as 'trouble' and likely to have behavioural problems without teachers looking deeper into possible causes.
>
> (Alexander-Passe 2015, p. 198)

It is easy to see how for some people, this can lead to frustration and eventually resentment, anger and even violent outbursts, with behaviours such as tyre slashing, criminal damage, graffiti, verbal abuse, muggings, etc. Such negative and resentful thoughts can lead to criminality, anti-social or anti-establishment behaviour, and feeling that this is the only way that they can ever achieve in the eyes of society, and the only way that they can attain more financial reward. This can result in theft, drug dealing, gang membership and generally mixing with a community where such behaviours are commonplace and even revered (Figure 6.1).

REFLECT ON THIS

Considering a global picture, how far do you believe that being able to read and write is a basic human right?

How far do you think that literacy is a mechanism for the pursuit of other human rights, such as a right to education, a right to access to health care etc.?

Prison population

There is an enormous amount of evidence from research that suggests that there is a disproportionate incidence of dyslexia among prison populations, not only in the UK but across the world (Kirk and Reid 1999; Reid and Kirk, 2001; Hunter-Carsch, 2001; Einat and Einat, 2008). These research studies show that between 30–50% of those in the criminal justice system in the UK are probably dyslexic. A similar position can be seen across the globe and a prestigious study by Alm and Andersson (1998) examined what they call penal institutions in Sweden and the USA, and found percentages as high as 45–65% of inmates with reading difficulties. Such weighty evidence does strongly link

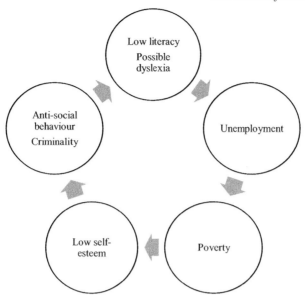

Figure 6.1 Cycle of anti-social behaviour and criminality

low levels of literacy and dyslexia to criminality; however, albeit a significant factor, it must only be seen as partly contributing to offending behaviour.

> A pattern of anti-social or maladjusted behavior at school might well lead to more serious forms of deviant behavior that end ultimately in imprisonment. If that pattern of behaviour was established it would not prove that dyslexia **caused** people to become delinquent: it would suggest that, if dyslexia is not carefully diagnosed and proper support provided, social disaffection might result. That is dyslexia might be shown to be indirectly related than directly related to offending behavior.
> (Reid and Kirk, 2001, p. 120; emphasis in original)

In 2005 Dyslexia Action investigated the links specifically between dyslexia and youth offending, they showed that 17.5% of the inmates in young offenders institutions were found to be dyslexic and between 84.5% and 87.6% were found to have low literacy skills (many of whom may have had undiagnosed dyslexia). Many in the sample had not been identified during their time in school but admitted to having been involved in low level anti-social behaviour prior to their convictions, including truancy, vehicle damage, joy riding, etc. As a consequence, the exact numbers with dyslexia and other information processing differences (IPDs) within the criminal justice system are hard to quantify. Recorded numbers have varied greatly depending upon the research project engaged with, but possibly also due to the criteria used to assess and identify. Some studies report as many as 52% of offenders with dyslexia and others only 31%, a difference of 21% which, at over one-fifth of the researched population, is a huge discrepancy, even at the lower level, between the often quoted 4–10% in the population as a whole.

With such large numbers being suggested there have been numerous attempts in the UK to research this further, such as the STOP project (Specific Training for Offenders on Probation) based in Shropshire, 1995–1997 (Davies and Byatt, 1998). This looked at the training, screening and assessment needs of young dyslexic offenders. This project attempted to devise a workable screening tool which was targeted specifically at young offenders; it recorded any difficulties with basic skills and any predisposing behavioural indicators of dyslexia, set within a real-life context. The STOP programme was designed to allow an assessment to be delivered by probation officers, who were non-specialists in dyslexia, but had received some basic training. Whilst this screening programme was not a definitive diagnosis of dyslexia, it aimed to identify those offenders at greatest risk and enabled referral to a fuller assessment in the future. Reid and Kirk (2001) reported the findings of the project which showed the following:

- 12% of the offenders tested were non-readers.
- 29% had such poor reading that finding employment in the future would likely be difficult.
- 24% were even unable to write their name reliably.
- 46% were unable to write simple text.
- 31% could be described as dyslexic or were exhibiting dyslexic tendencies.

This project attempted to be inclusive of numerous areas of the criminal justice system, believing that all those coming into contact with the young offenders needed to understand something of their difficulties. This would include:

- Probation officers
- Magistrates
- Police custody sergeants
- Volunteer mentors
- Employers
- Education staff
- Psychological training staff.

Another project that was around at this time was the Dyspel project (1995–1997). This was a study carried out by probation officers in London and reported on by Reid and Kirk (2001). This pilot project was set up to consider the training needs, support and awareness of dyslexia in those working with offenders, particularly the probation officers. It aimed to increase the number of offenders positively identified with dyslexic tendencies, and to consider the most appropriate specialist teaching programmes to reduce recidivism. Dyspel found that less than 5% of those identified with dyslexia whilst in prison had had their dyslexia identified during their time in school or education. The study showed that many had truanted from school or just did not attend, and some had attended specialist behavioural units. Almost all the identified inmates talked of very unhappy school days, of public humiliation, violence, frustration, bullying and mockery. They often had a complete lack of life direction and no belief that they could ever succeed at anything.

> Several spoke of standing outside colleges too frightened to go in, certain they would be told they were too stupid to get on a course.
> (Morgan and Klein, 2000, p. 60)

As a result of the Dyspel programme, a screening test was established which showed even higher levels of dyslexia among offenders than the STOP project.

This emphasis upon the link between dyslexia and offending, however often it has been found, is not universal, and a study by Rice (1998) and Rice et al. (2002), of 323 prisoners, showed no indication that dyslexia was disproportionately high in prisons and blamed the sampling measures and methodology used for the stark findings of the Dyspel project. There have been some critics of Rice (Reid and Kirk, 2001), which suggested that Rice used a poorly presented and outdated definition of dyslexia, which only considered criteria related to reading ability, thereby misrepresenting dyslexia as only an issue with literacy.

Examining the wealth of studies that have been undertaken in this area, the ones that do make links between dyslexia and criminality fall largely into two camps. Firstly, there are those such as Heiervang et al. (2001) that start with the premise that dyslexia is a neurological condition which correlates highly with criminal and anti-social behaviour. Secondly there is the camp that believes that dyslexia is a condition which, if not appropriately supported and managed by the educational establishment, can allow individuals to stray into the criminal fraternity.

Interview

Laura has three children, one with Asperger's and the other two are severely dyslexic and dyscalculic. She describes what happened with one of her sons starting in 1982.

> One of my boys, Ian, really found school difficult and could not understand what was happening there; he was always worried and 'on the edge'. Eventually we paid to see an educational psychologist as we were so worried, but this was not a good experience and he 'poo-pooed' the whole idea that my son was dyslexic or had anything wrong. My son began to self-harm, which was really distressing, he hated school so much

that he started to truant, which we were unaware of until the police became involved. His teachers were very professional, but they did not seem to understand dyslexia and claimed that it did not exist.

One night, when he was 16 years old, he got so drunk that we were called out to come and collect him from the police station, and we later found that he was also taking drugs. One night things got so bad that he went for me with a pair of scissors, it was really scary, as he did not seem to be aware of what was going on around him. My husband then asked him to leave home. He ended up living in one room of a house and on a number of occasions we had to raise money to bail him out of police custody. He needed to attend appointments with the police and probation service but frequently he was too disorganized and living on his own with no one to remind him, he would miss the appointments, which put him into more trouble. He did get jobs initially, but he was either made redundant or sacked from all of these.

My husband had a brain haemorrhage and we informed Ian, but there was no reaction from him, which was even more distressing. He had become very aggressive and to date he has been in prison three times for violence related offences.

Perhaps we should not have aspirations for our children? Perhaps we push them too far. We will always feel guilty for what has happened to Ian and blame ourselves. Neither my husband or myself is dyslexic, although my grandmother was left handed and I remember her telling us how she was forced to write with her right hand. In retrospect we would definitely have done things differently, but we are where we are and I cannot see a happy outcome for Ian.

Police

The difficulties experienced by those in the criminal justice system with dyslexia start long before they enter any sort of offender institution, and Morgan (1996) considered some of the issues that being processed by the police can have:

1. The police understandably have to place considerable emphasis on precise factual information, so when interviewing suspects, they expect a suspect or witness to have accurate recall of days, dates and times. This can be extremely difficult for someone with dyslexia who is likely to have sequential memory difficulties. Remembering things in the correct order and the succession of events can be very challenging for all people when under the stress of a police interview, but particularly so for those with an IPD. On the positive side however, the tendency for those with dyslexia to have a more holistic thinking pattern can make their role as a witness very useful, as they will often be able to 'see' the events in a more global picture, and remember things that others may not.

2   Any visit to a police station, no matter for what reason, even for lost property or a stray dog, always requires the participant to fill in a plethora of forms. For someone accused of a felony, of any sort, they will be required to read extensive documents, often in legalized jargon, which can be extremely challenging. For many with low literacy, this means signing a document without reading it first and this can mean signing away certain rights that we would normally expect to have. They may be unaware of their rights, particularly to legal representation, or even how to access volunteer assistance with their reading. In many cases the shame of being unable to read is often too great for them to inform those who are processing their case.
3   Another area that can prove difficult is the requirement to attend a series of court appearances or interviews with their legal representatives. To miss a court appearance is viewed as a serious offence and can have significant consequences upon any subsequent sentencing. For someone who has genuine difficulties remembering times and dates, this can be confusing and disastrous, unless they have a supportive family member or mentor, who can keep track of these appointments and add reminders for them.
4   Finally, when the accused finally appears in court, they are frequently asked to read material and even to read out loud, a very frightening experience for anyone attending the formality of court proceedings, but particularly so for someone with an IPD. The embarrassment, shame and even fear that they feel is acute, and for many is the hardest part of the whole ordeal, but admitting to their condition is often too painful to be possible.

Interview: appropriate adult (acting as advocate) in the criminal justice system

> Despite the common-sense belief that people do not confess to crimes they did not commit, 20 to 25% of all DNA exonerations involve innocent prisoners who confessed.
>
> (Kassin, 2008, p. 249)

> As to what makes juveniles so vulnerable, developmental research indicates that adolescents display an 'immaturity of judgment' in their decision making – a pattern of behavior that is characterized by impulsivity, a focus on immediate gratification, and a diminished capacity for perceptions of future risk.
>
> (Kassin 2008, p. 251)

The role of an appropriate adult (henceforth referred to as AA) is to ensure that the person arrested understands their rights and reads all the material to them when there is no family support member available. The AA ensures that they are treated fairly. Under the Police and Criminal Evidence Act 1984 (PACE) Codes of Practice, police custody sergeants must secure an AA (who may be a friend or family member), to safeguard the rights and welfare of vulnerable people detained or questioned by the police. This is a critical safeguard to the justice system that arose in part due to the number of vulnerable people confessing to crimes they did not commit.

Jenny is a volunteer and trained as an AA to work with under eighteen-year-olds and vulnerable adults who have been arrested and taken into custody.

> A very high percentage of those I work with have literacy issues, I would estimate approximately 85%. Some are only able to write their first name and are unable to complete an appropriate signature. Many find it hard to understand the language, even conversational language, even when their first language is English.
>
> I would estimate that approximately half of those with literacy problems are dyslexic and have received that identification at some point in their lives.
>
> The police service is usually extremely good, and they call for the appropriate adult to attend and support the arrestee, although some are perhaps not as sympathetic or understanding of the difficulties being experienced by the arrestee. They do not understand that they may have more difficulties than just reading problems.
>
> None of the arrestees that I have attended have been employed, and most live in either supported living accommodation or are of no fixed abode. Most of them are single.
>
> Often there are other co-morbid conditions such as ADHD [attention deficit and hyperactivity disorder], ADD [Attention deficit disorder], Asperger's etc.
>
> The sort of offences committed are:
>
> - Illegal drugs possession and dealing
> - Wielding knives and offensive weapons
> - Actual bodily harm
> - Criminal damage
> - Disorder
> - Attempted murder
> - Murder/manslaughter.
>
> So, the nature of the offences is very wide, from petty criminals to much more serious offences. I have only had to sit with one arrestee for more than one occasion, but it is clear that many of them are repeat offenders from the conversations that the police are having with them. Several have already had custodial sentences.
>
> I feel that there is a general lack of support in society, even in the supported accommodation, especially when they leave school. I believe that most are not hardened criminals but are in the wrong place, and it becomes a vicious circle with their low self-esteem. They need somewhere else to go other than the criminal justice system, and above all they need to be shown how to read, even in a rudimentary way.
>
> They are usually very grateful to me for acting as their appropriate adult and appreciate the support especially from someone not in uniform.

Models of criminality

Traditionally there are three fundamental models of criminality:

1 The psychological model: this starts with the premise that our personality drives our behaviours, and the criminal behaviour stems from a deviance or dysfunction within the development of our personality. This is based on a largely Freudian approach, believing that early childhood experiences are at the heart of our personality development, and these experiences can increase our impulsivity, reduce our capacity for empathy and inhibit normal feeling of guilt.
2 The biological model: this implies that we are either born with an inherent flaw in our biological make up, or the flaw comes as a result of a trauma. In the past this theory has resulted in some quite drastic surgery, including lobotomies, or chemical interventions such as the use of Ritalin for those identified with ADD/ADHD, to 'correct' the flaws.
3 The social model: this attempts to connect criminality to broad social structures within society and views on morality within cultures. Durkheim (1897) related this to feeling disconnected from society which could result in a loss of aspiration to achieve, and unequal opportunities between groups, often but not always, related to poverty.

There is no reason to suppose that these are distinct and separate categories, and probably the truth is more about a close interweaving of these three models. Being dyslexic does not automatically mean that an individual is going to follow a criminal pathway, and there is unlikely to be one reason, or one distinct model, that can indicate why one does and another does not. Way back in 1968 Critchley emphasised that this link to crime was the greatest in those who were previously unidentified with dyslexia (the undiagnosed dyslexia), and this has been reiterated by many subsequent research projects (Kirk and Reid, 1999; Dyslexia Action 2005; Macdonald, 2010).

> The link between dyslexia and crime in fact relates not to people diagnosed with the condition, but to people with undiagnosed dyslexia.
> (Macdonald, 2010, p. 2010)

According to Macdonald (2010) there are three categories of individuals with dyslexia:

1 Those with the most severe dyslexia who show all the classical signs and find that they cannot function effectively in the mainstream education system. It could be suggested that this is the most fortunate group, as they are so starkly different from their peers that this group is highly likely to be identified and offered appropriate support for their differences. This often occurs at a very early age and the support can be appropriately tailored to their particular needs.

2   The second group are highly likely to be unidentified dyslexics, or at least not identified until much later in their educational career. Macdonald (2010) suggests that this is probably the largest group and they are often highly skilled at concealing the difficulties they experience.
3   Finally, there is the group that are never identified, or at least not until later adult life. Macdonald (2010) believes that this is the group most likely to experience the most difficulties.

In the research undertaken by Macdonald (2010) into links between crime and dyslexia, none of the sample of previously undiagnosed prison *inmates* had been employed for at least a year prior to being incarcerated, and many had been living off state funded benefits for many years, some since leaving school. It is likely that their low literacy contributed to their inability to gain employment; this is further exacerbated when they commit offences and receive a criminal record. Often the offences committed related to financial gain, in the mistaken belief that this could relieve the poverty that they found themselves in. Macdonald (2010) reported that once in the system and identified as having an IPD, they gained access to educational support, many going on to gain formal qualifications, which could improve their chances of employability upon release. Offenders reported that this made huge differences to their lives, and Macdonald (2010) reported that their employment rates went up by as much as 55%, making not only a difference to their economic circumstances, but, probably even more importantly, to their self-esteem and confidence.

Disabling barriers

Disabling barriers is a term used when the society in which you live does not cater for your particular needs. Barricades are put up by society, not necessarily intentionally, to prevent those with disabilities from fully participating. Such barriers are often not fully recognised by the non-disabled community, and most people would be upset to realise that they were there. Such barriers, however unintentional, help to marginalise and segregate those with physical and cognitive differences, as they are imposed upon them by society. The barriers can differ widely and the impact that they have upon people will also vary widely, depending upon the needs of that individual. Examples of such barriers may fall into certain categories:

1   Physical barriers: this might be limiting access to places, either through the physical environment, steps instead of ramps, narrow entrances and exits, unsuitable chairs and furniture, but could also be related to expense, for example suitable transport too costly to allow access to leisure and employment.
2   Language barriers: this might refer to the language used to talk about people with disabilities and their negative connotations, creating stigma and in some cases fear.

3   Cultural and psychological barriers: in some cultures, disability is seen as a curse or evil spirit; some conditions, such as dyslexia, are not always recognised and even actively denied.
4   Societal structures and accepted norms as barriers: issues of gender, ethnicity religion and societal attitudes towards these groups of people.
5   Political barriers: that is policies, procedures and situations that systematically disadvantage those with disabilities, such as welfare and the benefit system, finance allocations to education and the health service resources, etc.

Such barriers can create situations in which individuals experience social exclusion, and become detached from society and the places that they live and work. This in turn can result in a low quality of life, poor employment prospects and poor living accommodation.

Socio-economic aspects and poverty

Research by Macdonald (2009) indicated that not only are disabling barriers such as dyslexia impeding education and employment opportunities for these individuals, but this is further exacerbated by levels of socio-economic status.

People from low socio-economic backgrounds experience far more disabling barriers, owing to the lack of economic and social capital, than their middle-class counterparts:

> working class dyslexic participants in this study found it more difficult to overcome their literacy restrictions and gain employment within adulthood, than middle-class dyslexic participants.
> (Macdonald, 2010, p. 35)

Macdonald (2010), implies that poverty and social status strongly impact on individuals experience of dyslexia and the social inequalities of society. It could be surmised that those who have limited financial backing cannot afford to pay for the sort of assistive technology, physical resources, expert support assistance and assessments that those with more disposable income can afford. Macdonald (2010) believes that this link between dyslexia and poverty is fundamental to the link between dyslexia and criminality (Figure 6.2).

Criminality and normality

If *most* people do something, society tends to regard it as 'normal'. West (1982) reminds us that most, if not all, people exhibit anti-social behaviour and even criminality, therefore it should be regarded as 'normal'. We all commit crime from time to time: exceeding the speed limit, dropping litter, even theft. How many of us can truthfully say that we have always informed a shop assistant when they have undercharged us for an item, or as a child have not helped ourselves to extra sweets

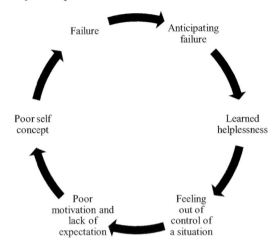

Figure 6.2 The cycle of failure

and goodies from the shop, or have not hiked up an insurance claim? How many of us have not lied to get out of paying a parking fine, or 'bunking off' school? West (1982) suggests that society sees youth offending as in some way different to 'real' offending, blaming their lack of understanding of right and wrong on a poor upbringing. Society appears to accept that it is about degree and not the criminal act itself, it is okay to steal a few sweets but not to rob a bank, okay to defraud a large insurance company but not a little old lady!

West (1982) suggests that the idea of crime and anti-social behaviour being 'normal' and only about degree needs to be questioned, and attributes these attitudes to a variety of criteria linked to childhood.

1 Psychological and personality differences
2 Family history of criminality: growing up in an environment with family dynamics where criminality is accepted
3 Socio-cultural inequalities
4 Lack of education and institutional failure
5 Opportunities for such conduct and learned behaviour
6 Peer group culture and pressure
7 Socio-economic factors and unemployment
8 Levels of isolation and segregation.

Supportive other

One theme that appears to run throughout the stories of dyslexia is the importance of someone who is supportive and understanding. This could be a family member, but not always, and could be a friend, an employer, a teacher or other professional. For those not lucky enough to have stumbled across that supportive *other* their story can be of a very negative and downward spiralling nature. Research has repeatedly shown (Morgan, 1996: Kirk and Reid, 2000; Hewitt-Main, 2012) that there is a disproportionate number of individuals with an IPD in the criminal justice system, but there appears to be no evidence that having a learning difference genetically predisposes someone to take a socially deviant pathway through life, so it is reasonable to surmise that this is environmentally constructed.

Hewitt-Main (2012) undertook a project of education and mentoring in Chelmsford prison which appeared to demonstrate some spectacular results. Inmates were offered educational opportunities with close mentoring; to begin with this was mentoring from the professionals, but as the project progressed inmates who had been engaging with the system were trained to teach and mentor fellow inmates. At the start of the project 60% of the prisoners opted out of either work or training, and as they later revealed, this was for fear of revealing their low literacy skills and a fear of classrooms and schools.

> Many prisoners [at Chelmsford] complained of the difficulties of going straight because even building work required the passing of a basic test and almost everything required the filling in of application forms or passing theory tests. They couldn't even apply for benefits without admitting they need help.
> (Hewitt-Main, 2012, p. 7)

The results of the mentoring programme were transformational, according to Hewitt-Main (2012), with prison officers claiming that the prison overall was calmer, and even the most violent prisoners less volatile as their self-esteem rose. Altogether the prison at Chelmsford became a happier place requiring less intervention from the prison staff. This project demonstrated a significant reduction in reoffending rates, albeit this was a small sample, but after four years only one prisoner had been returned to the criminal justice system, that is 5.9% recidivism, compared with the government accepted 55–68% (Hewitt-Main, 2012). If this rate could be replicated across the criminal justice system Hewitt-Main (2012) claims that there are potentially huge savings of taxpayers' money, running to billions of pounds. If each prisoner costs the tax payer £100,000 per annum to keep, (including police, court appearances, probation, state funding for families, etc.), as estimated by Hewitt-Main (2012), such literacy mentoring projects could save the government and the taxpayer eye-watering sums of money, make the general community safer and the prisons and young offenders institutions calmer and less aggressive places to work and live. According to the UK Government statistics in 2017, the prison population was 874,746 and rising (Gov UK, 2017).

REFLECT ON THIS

Use the following questions to discuss with a colleague or in a staff meeting:

1 Some disabling barriers have been highlighted in this chapter, can you think of any more and how could these be overcome?

2   Can the issue of stigma be overcome by abandoning the labelling process?
3   If the education system had sufficient funds and expertise to identify and support all children at risk of an IPD, would fewer end up in the criminal justice system, or would prisons still be full to capacity?
4   Would better identification and support for dyslexia lead to fewer mental health issues in society?

Interview

Wanda is head of inclusion at a large male prison facility. She works for an organisation that delivers education and training to adults and young people in UK prisons and young offenders' institutions. The stated aim of the organisation is to reduce reoffending rates. Wanda has worked at the prison for one year, but previously spent several years working with young offenders in another part of the country. She has had considerable success with the young offenders, and has been brought into the prison to replicate that success.

> One of the biggest differences in the young offenders' institution and the prison is the funding. As a young offender you are entitled to education in the same way as you would if you went to a state funded school or college. As an adult prisoner no such funding is available, there is some draw down money, but this is very limited.
>
> The young offenders who are identified with special needs are given an EHC plan [education, health and care plan], they are assessed by a specialist within the institution and up to the age of 25 years of age can access funding for support. In the prison no such system exists, and there are no specialist assessors that I can refer residents to, so there is no diagnosis for dyslexia made in the prison. There is no one with the special knowledge and skills to refer residents to.
>
> We have devised our own questionnaire, which we use to help to identify at risk residents, and we are currently exploring the possibility of a computer based model of the assessment.
>
> [Interviewer] What do you see in the prisoners that you work with?
>
> I see a cycle of parents with low literacy having children who also find it hard to read and write … it appears normal in their homes, most have dropped out of school and once they go into the outside world they talk about having no confidence and feeling shame. Most have no self-worth, and most are unemployed, often because they cannot apply for a job.
>
> Some of them are self-declarers and some are proud to be able to say that they find reading and writing difficult, but that is because they are dyslexic … it is almost as though they are saying 'I am not stupid … I have a label'!
>
> The residents we do help are helped through a Sharon Trust reading plan [Sharon Trust is a charitable organisation that supports up to 4,000 prisoners to learn to read and write through a peer to peer mentoring system], other residents, who are confident readers, are trained to work with non-readers as a mentor and a friend.

[Interviewer] Do you have any particular philosophy when working with your residents?

Yes. I do not believe in labels, we always work with the whole person and not with the behaviour, better that you define that person's way of working and adapt your teaching to that, then it is important to articulate that to everyone that works with that resident. We try to look at the person and why they are doing what they are doing.

I believe in the whole concept of neurodiversity, which is why it is so important to differentiate your teaching methods and strategies to ensure that they are dyslexia friendly. We use coloured paper and ensure a readable font that the resident is comfortable with. Even the PowerPoint presentations and overlays that we use are appropriately coloured.

Unfortunately, because of the nature of the prison environment residents are not allowed to use laptop computers or assistive technology, so programmes such as Dragon Naturally, which would be really helpful, are not available to us.

[Interviewer] What sort of response do you get from your residents?

Generally, the response is brilliant, and they really understand that we are there to help them. Of course, we do encounter resistance and frustration at times, but aggression is very rare.

Learners can access all levels of education from level one to an Open University Degree. Clearly there is still work to be done but we do have an excellent success rate.

[Interviewer] What about the other prison staff?

The prison officers are really good, but they sometimes do not appear to be aware of the whole person. Their initial training is centred around prison craft and security and it would be good if they could be made more aware of dyslexia and low literacy, when they are first training for the job. Occasionally I have been approached by an officer who self-declares that he has a problem with literacy and asks to join in with the programme.

Chapter reflections

The logical conclusion of this chapter is to improve the identification and available support within the education system and to reduce the offending and reoffending behaviour of those with dyslexia, by recognising their condition at an early age and ensuring that appropriate and research based support and technology are in place. The reasoning behind this is to prevent the disaffection and low grade anti-social behaviour developing and evolving into full blown criminality. Much greater support for literacy learning in offender institutions is required but that support needs to continue beyond the institutions and upon release, possibly through the probation service and supported voluntary organisations. These issues have implications for professionals and volunteers in the criminal justice system, but also for politicians relating to schools, education and staff training.

Although the cycle of offending is a complex matter, literacy skills are recognized as a key factor in reducing and breaking these cycles of crime.
(Macdonald, 2010, p. 52)

This chapter is very much a snapshot of the wealth of research and expert opinion that has gone into the reasons behind criminal behaviour. Such a complex psychological and sociological approach cannot be explored within the confines of this chapter, but it can indicate some of the thinking from the many research projects behind this multifaceted area, and possible associations with IPDs as a pathway to crime.

Further reading

Macdonald, SJ (2010) *Crime and Dyslexia: A Social Model Approach*. Berlin: Deutsche Nationalbiblothek.

This very readable text examines a social model of dyslexia and its relationship with crime, going beyond the more established educational view of dyslexia. Macdonald rejects any form of biological/medical model which suggests that those with dyslexia are inherently more likely to commit antisocial behaviour and criminal acts, and examines the role that society and structural inequalities play.

Macdonald uses his examination of the available research to show that social organisation and society provide inclusive and exclusive networks, leading to the creation of social barriers to those with cognitive and neurological differences. He examines the psycho-social explanations for criminal behaviour, in both Europe and the USA, and how relative poverty and socio-economic disparities can lead to criminality.

In this book are the results of qualitative and quantitative primary research, conducted by Macdonald, examining the risk factors that underpin criminality and the cycle of low literacy, poverty and anti-social behaviour.

References

Alexander-Passe, N (2015) *Dyslexia and Mental Health*. London: Jessica Kingsley.
Alm, J and Andersson, J (1998) *The Dyslexia Project at the Employability Institute of Uppsala*. Gnesta, Sweden: Swedish National Labour Board.
Critchley, M (1968) Reading retardation, dyslexia and delinquency. *The British Journal of Psychiatry* 114: 1537–1547.
Davies, K and Byatt, J (1998) *Something Can be Done!* Shrewsbury: Shropshire STOP Project.
Durkheim, E (1897) [1951 translation] *Suicide: A Study in Sociology*. Paris: The Free Press.
Dyslexia Action (2005) *The Hidden Disabilities in the Prison Population*. Surrey: The Dyslexia Institute.
Einat, T and Einat, A (2008) Learning disabilities and delinquency: a study of Israeli prison inmates. *International Journal of Offender Therapy and Comparative Criminology* 52 (4): 416–434.

Gov UK (2017) *Prison Population Figures: 2017.* www.gov.uk/government/statistics/prison-population-figures-2017 (accessed 28. 11. 19).

Heiervang, E, Stevenson, J, Lund, A and Hugdahl, K (2001) Behaviour problems in children with dyslexia. *Nordic Journal of Psychiatry* 55(4): 251–256.

Hewitt-Main, J (2012) *Dyslexia Behind Bars: Final Report of Pioneering Teaching and Mentoring Project at Chelmsford Prison, 4 Years On.* Chelmsford: Mentoring4U.

Hunter-Carsch, M (2001) *Dyslexia: A Psychosocial Perspective.* London: Whurr.

Kassin, SM (2008) False confessions: causes, consequences and implications for reform. *Current Direction in Psychological Science* 17(4): 249–253.

Kirk, J and Reid, G (1999) *Adult Dyslexia for Employment and Training (ADEPT).* Edinburgh: University of Edinburgh.

Kirk, J and Reid, G (2001) An examination of the relationship between dyslexia and offending in young people and the implications for the training system. *Dyslexia* 7(2): 77–84.

Kirk, J and Reid, G (2003) *Adult Dyslexia Checklist: Criteria and considerations.* BDA Handbook. Reading: BDA.

Macdonald, SJ (2009) *Towards a Sociology of Dyslexia: Exploring the Links Between Dyslexia, Disability and Social Class.* Saarbrücken: VDM Publishing House Ltd.

Macdonald, SJ (2010) *Crime and Dyslexia: A Social Model Approach.* Berlin: Deutsche Nationalbiblothek.

Morgan, E and Klein, C (2000) *The Dyslexic Adult in a Non-Dyslexic World.* London: Whurr Publications.

Morgan W (1996) Dyslexic offenders. *The Magistrate Magazine* 52(4): 84–86.

Reid, G and Kirk, J (2001) *Dyslexia in Adults: Education and Employment.* Chichester: John Wiley.

Rice, M (1998) *Dyslexia and Crime: Some Notes on the Dyspel Claim.* Cambridge: University of Cambridge, Institute of Criminology.

Rice, M, Howes, M and Connel, P (2002) *The Prison Reading Survey: A Report to HM Prison Service Planning Group.* Cambridge: University of Cambridge, Institute of Criminology.

Saunders C (1990) Dyslexia as a factor in the young adult offender. In Hales, G (ed) *Meeting Points in Dyslexia.* Reading: BDA.

West, D (1982) *Delinquency, Its Roots, Career and Prospects.* London: Heinemann.

7 Employment
Cost to employers/employees

> We know what we are, but not what we may be.
> (William Shakespeare, *Hamlet. Prince of Denmark*, Act 4 Scene 5, p. 872)

Introduction

The British Dyslexia Association (BDA) (2019) estimates that there are up to 2.9 million workers affected by information processing differences (IPDs). It is therefore vital that employers develop a satisfactory understanding of dyslexia beyond the generally recognised literacy difficulties. It is intended that this chapter will examine the reasons behind the reluctance that many people have to disclose their dyslexia, perhaps fearing that in the harsh reality of the labour market they may become victimised, and that employers may be unsympathetic to their needs. This chapter will analyse issues behind providing mentoring and safe confidential spaces for disclosure and decision making, within the legal confines of the Equality Act 2010.

Employability

One of the great strengths that some people with dyslexia possess is a very different way of thinking, the whole 'big picture thinking', the ability to see patterns and manipulate shapes and ideas in the mind, inventiveness and creativity. In fact, these are often the very skills which employers value most, and are often the reason why so many of our brilliant inventions and artistic creations have come from people with IPDs, such as Leonardo da Vinci, Pablo Picasso, Benjamin Zephaniah, Carly Simon, etc. Entrepreneurs such as Sir Richard Branson, Jamie Oliver and Sir Alan Sugar have all disclosed that they have an IPD. Such artistic and creative skills have served man well over thousands of years, and probably are the reason why Homo sapiens have survived and controversially risen to the top of the animal kingdom. The strengths that many with IPDs are likely to have were probably a significant evolutionary advantage, that is until the invention of the written word, which does not suit this particular way of thinking. Only when reading and writing became such a vital component of human life did those with IPDs begin to struggle, and for these conditions to be seen as disabilities rather than abilities.

In the twenty-first century most job roles require the applicant to be able to read and write: even physical manual work requires the reading of job sheets, job completion forms, timesheets, taxation forms and the ability to manipulate numbers and letters. Most job roles now require training, qualifications and certificates.

> Jobs that allow flexibility can open the door to success for dyslexics. It's often while devising new methods for routine tasks that dyslexics come up with innovative approaches that save time, effort and expense and improve outcomes for everyone.
>
> (Eide and Eide, 2011, p. 240)

Eide and Eide (2011) suggest that to be successful in employment an individual with dyslexia must be allowed flexibility, and the opportunity for creativity and innovation. They believe that this is more difficult to achieve in a large corporation which relies on uniformity of rules and rigid systems, than in a small working environment where each employee is known to the employer. For many with an IPD the lack of suitable employment, due to that rigidity of systems and intolerance of diverse thinking styles, causes many with dyslexia to find employment in small or start-up companies, which are likely to value more innovative ways of working, and be more agreeable to 'out-of-the-box' thinking. For many the answer to employment is to start up their own business, and according to Eide and Eide (2011) the number of entrepreneurs with an IPD is disproportionately high compared with the general population.

Logan (2009) quotes a figure of only 1% of middle managers in large corporations having an IPD, but this figure could be considerably higher in senior management positions. Logan's research showed that 35% of entrepreneurs in America reported dyslexic traits compared to a national American average of 15%, which was found to be considerably higher than in the UK, although Logan (2009) provides no appropriate explanation for their difference.

Education to workplace

The transition from school and education to the workplace is always a profound experience, no matter who you are. This experience can be both positive and negative but can be particularly challenging for someone with an IPD. Education is driven by teachers and experts in particular areas of knowledge; they accept that their students will be making mistakes during their learning experiences, and will often use these as opportunities for learning, to be worked with and developed. Driven by government funding and inspection reports, exams become a focal target of the curriculum which is often totally arranged around the need to achieve certain grades and standards to access particular areas of employment or further and higher education. In schools, colleges and universities, pastoral care of their students and pupils is frequently claimed to be an important area of their work. We expect teachers to understand that children cannot learn what they want to teach, if they are in emotional turmoil. In 2015 the then Schools Minister the Rt Hon Nick Gibb addressed the Education Reform Summit and claimed that in the eyes of the government of the day the purpose of education is:

> [as an] engine of our economy; it is the foundation of our culture and it is an essential preparation for adult life.
>
> (Gibb, 2015)

He continued by saying that the aim of education is to provide greater social justice and a fairer society. In short, schools and education focused upon the individual and developing the individual for their future life, but students know that this is a very temporary phase in their lives (maybe only two or three years), and they are usually very aware of the end date. However, in the world of work the focus is very different, here the attention is upon the workplace and not the individual (of course these are very broad generalisations but are indicative of a general culture). In schools there will be large numbers of inexperienced individuals and only a very few who are experienced and knowledgeable in the field, but in the workplace the balance and the dynamics are very different; often there are very many experienced and much older people, with only a few who are inexperienced, novices and apprentices. Many of the experienced workers in a working environment have been there for many years, for some all their working lives. These people have an absolute grasp of the roles they assume and the tasks they are asked to perform. In the workplace most people will not be working on the same task at the same time, as they might in education, but each individual may be performing different tasks, although they may rely upon the others to complete their tasks before bringing together an overall production. Some will have demanding and complex tasks to achieve, others will have less complex but equally demanding tasks, in a very different way. Errors in the workplace are not seen as learning experiences, as they are in education, but rather as major issues which could result in huge financial implications to the company and reprimand, or even dismissal, by line managers. Losing one's job means a lack of employment, which could in turn bring financial challenges to the individual which could have long reaching consequences to family lives, housing and lifestyle.

Fitzgibbon and O'Connor (2002) discuss the difference between the types of learning in education and the typical training promoted in the workplace. The biggest difference, they suggest, is that in education the learning is generalised, to enable the student to apply this learning to many differing situations; however in workplace training it is usually very focused upon a particular task or area of expertise, and is usually *practical and concrete* (Fitzgibbon and O'Connor, 2002, p. 34). They also point out that the pace of learning is different, usually being more relaxed in schools, with students able to explore and investigate an area, but in the workplace the training needs to be focused and delivered quickly with strict deadlines, usually related exclusively to that particular workplace. The emphasis in education is upon individuals researching the knowledge, learning through a process, but in the workplace, the trainer presents the material for immediate consumption with no requirement or expectation that the trainee will question or critique that learning.

For those with an IPD even the first day in their new job role can be challenging; Table 7.1 lists some of the difficulties identified by those interviewed for this text.

In a report written for the TUC in 2014, Hagan suggested that employees with dyslexia are more likely to experience disciplinary and misconduct problems than those without, and these issues appeared to be directly related to their disability. Hagan (2014) also indicates that those with dyslexia report high levels of bullying and stress, which he believes are attributable to ignorance of the condition on the part of management and colleagues, therefore serious mismanagement of the situation is possible.

Owning up

Dyslexia is often described as a hidden disability, which means that from the outside it is impossible to tell who has an IPD and who does not, unlike a physical disability which is likely to be very apparent. This means that if an employer is to know whether their employee or potential recruit has an IPD, the individual needs to self-declare. This can only be done if the individual themselves already knows that they have such a condition, which many do not. As can be seen in a number of the interviews conducted for this book, such self-declaration can become a huge dilemma and complex decisions need to be made, such as:

1   Whether to inform an employer at the time of the recruitment process, and risk not being considered for the role, due to a possible misunderstanding or ignorance of the condition by the recruiters/employers.

Table 7.1 Common difficulties in the workplace

Getting lost	Interviews	Completing order forms
Filling in application forms	Verbal presentations	Completing expenses claims forms
Filling in record cards/forms	Undertaking performance reviews	Keeping financial data accurate, such a travel expenses, etc.
Planning and sequencing	Time management	Interpreting pay slips
Completing tax forms	Promotion procedures	Keeping accurate diaries
Attending meetings on time	Slow to perform certain tasks	Data management

2 Whether to inform the employer after their appointment, which could be seen to have serious ethical implications.
3 Whether to deliberately conceal (even lie), and risk being 'found out' at a later stage, knowing that they will have to forego the accommodations that they are legally entitled to. This type of concealment by non-disclosure is sometimes excused by saying *no one asked me*!
4 Whether to disclose in part, and be selective in the information revealed, holding back issues that might be a problem in that particular appointment.

With so much riding upon this disclosure, it is not surprising that many simply withhold the information for fear of victimisation, and put in place their own strategies for overcoming their difficulties, as they probably have throughout their schooling and education, despite the Equality Act 2010, which should protect against discrimination because of disability. However, it must be remembered that an employer only has an obligation under the Equality Act 2010 if they know, or ought reasonably to know, that their employee has a disability.

Vogel and Adelman (2000) studied self-disclosure in adults with dyslexia and showed that 41% of those studied did not want to reveal to their employers that they were dyslexic. These individuals probably thought that there was a risk factor to self-disclosure which they were not ready to take, even when they were aware of the adjustments that could be made for them, or they could feel too embarrassed; some of those interviewed for this book told me: *It's none of their business!*

> In an ideal world, individuals would never need to conceal their dyslexia, because their employers and co-workers would understand ... that dyslexia is associated with strengths as well as challenges and individuals with dyslexia have abilities that can be useful in almost any kind of job. Unfortunately, our world hasn't yet reached that ideal state and ignorance keeps some employers wary of giving individuals with dyslexia a chance to prove their worth.
>
> (Eide and Eide, 2011, p. 247)

Dale and Aiken (2007) made a study of nurses within the National Health Service, who were aware of their dyslexia, but who worked hard to conceal this from their colleagues and line managers, for fear of discrimination. Many of the nurses believed that the risk to their career and the stigma which could ensue were too great to disclose and were therefore unable to access the accommodations that they were entitled to.

Because dyslexia is a hidden disability it is likely to be less well understood by the general public, so the importance of self-advocacy cannot be overemphasised. However, both self-disclosure and self-advocacy are very personal issues, and almost certainly some people will wish for it to remain private, and there is no legal obligation for them to disclose. Self-disclosure must be the right choice for the individual at the right time, and be approached in their own way.

> If the dyslexic does not disclose their disability, then they can get into all sorts of trouble because there is no good explanation when things go wrong. Disorganisation and poor memory can lead to disasters that can look like incompetence, carelessness or an inability to do the job.
>
> (Scott, 2004, p. 231)

Research for this book confirms Scott's (2004) claim that there is very little evidence for research into the rates of disclosure in the UK, but he predicted this to be as low as 2%; however, in the USA disclosure rates are thought to be at 20% although he offers no explanation of why that might be. Whether an employee with disclosed dyslexia gets the support in their workplace to which they are entitled is very hit and miss according to Hoffmann et al. (1987) and is probably extremely low. Hoffmann et al. (1987) also showed in their research that only 24% of employers made appropriate modifications to the workplace for those who disclosed dyslexia although this may have improved since the research by Hoffmann et al., with the introduction of the Equality Act 2010, but research in this area appears limited.

> Section 60 of the Equality Act 2010 outlines areas where an employer may reasonably require information about a disability – either at a job application or promotion review; it may well be problematic for an employee who withholds this information if asked, but subsequently seeks to rely on the Act's other positive provisions.
>
> (Hagan, 2014, p. 10)

Reasonable adjustments

Legally an employer is bound by the Equality Act 2010, which states that an employer must not discriminate against someone with a disability: dyslexia is a recognised disability under the Equality Act 2010 and employers are bound to make reasonable adjustments to their premises and practices to accommodate such a disability. Failure to make such adjustments could count as unlawful discrimination and they could be subject to an employment tribunal. However, making reasonable adjustments under the Equality Act 2010 means going further than just unfavourable treatment, but means taking positive action. The Equality and Human Rights Commission (2016) states that reasonable adjustments must be made and must not be taken as a reason for impeding appropriate promotion of a worker with a disability or be a reason to dismiss or suspend a worker. However, employers are not legally required to employ someone who cannot do the job, but where that person is the best fit for the job, then they *are* required to make accommodations for that. This may mean being responsible for arranging and covering the costs of a full diagnostic workplace needs assessment, as part of their commitment to reasonable adjustment. In reality the expense of this may (unlawfully) deter an employer from taking on a worker with a disability, fearing that it will be costly and difficult.

The term *reasonable adjustment* is readily bandied about, but it is not always so easy to define. Employers are not always sure what this means; previous chapters of this book have shown that there is a generalised mistaken belief that dyslexia is only about reading, writing and literacy and anyone with an IPD must understand that the likelihood is that many employers will fall into this category of people. Most employers will not have specialist knowledge of the condition, and undoubtedly some or even many will believe that those with dyslexia simply cannot read and write at all. This lack of understanding of the condition by employers means that they are unlikely to understand that with some very small adaptations to the workplace the dyslexic adult can become a valuable and innovative member of their team. However, this is a two-way street and, in reality, adaptations probably need to be made on both sides, employee and employer. Some will query what the term 'reasonable' means: this is a word that can have many connotations and may vary according to the individual using it, and their circumstances. Understandably employers are going to be concerned what such adjustments are going to cost them, both financially and in practical, reorganisational terms, but in reality, many are very easy to implement and do not cost a great deal. When the adjustments required do become more costly, such as a Workplace Needs Assessment (WNA), to determine what adjustments are required or particular pieces of technological hardware or software, it is sometimes possible to offset some of this against taxation or to gain full or part financial assistance from the government, under the Department for Work and Pensions, Access to Work scheme.

The Department of Health states that a reasonable adjustment is:

> An adjustment to the workplace or work practice that is effective for the employee without being too disruptive, costly or impractical for the employer to provide.
>
> (DoH, 2019)

However, this definition is very 'woolly' and the term *too costly* is variable and may differ if the employer is a large multinational conglomerate or a small, but expanding, one-man business. However, Beetham (2018) reminds us that a *reasonable adjustment* is not just a 'nice to have' but a 'must have' for people with any disability, and without these employers may not be getting as much as they could from that employee, as they will probably not be working to their full potential and not bringing the creative flair and innovation to the workplace that many with that 'out-of-the-box' type thinking often can do. This, in turn, can lead to stress for the employee and even mental and physical health issues.

Before employing anyone with a disability and implementing any reasonable adjustments an employer will need to consider a number of things:

1. Whether the adjustments implemented will significantly help their employee and ensure that they are not disadvantaged by their disability and therefore help their business to grow and thrive.
2. Whether the change to the working environment is likely to be too disruptive, for example using voicemail rather than email could be a problem for customers of that business and other employees.
3. Whether the cost of the adjustments outweigh the benefits, for example having a Workplace Needs Assessment (WNA) may cost £400–£600 plus, possible voice recognition software and text-to-speech and digital recorders for meetings, a further £100–£500 and whether there is external funding readily available to assist with this.
4. Whether the organisation already has appropriate resources, which they could make available. A small employer with only one or two employees clearly is less likely to have the resources or experience available to it than a large employer with hundreds of employees and a specially designated equal opportunities and human resources department.

Hagan (2014), writing in a report for the TUC, suggests that misunderstandings by employers of what constitutes reasonable adjustment under the Equality Act 2010 also places a heavy load upon employees. Employers need to be aware that, according to the TUC (Hagan, 2014), there is no cap on the levels of compensation that can be claimed by someone with dyslexia if they go on to prove, in a tribunal, that discrimination has occurred in the workplace. A tribunal will consider this carefully on a case-by-case basis before making judgement and, even for the successful complainant, this may not result in what they want most, and that is lasting and fulfilling employment.

Fitzgibbon and O'Connor (2002) suggest that many with dyslexia find it unnecessarily stressful in the workplace because they are not given 'the tools they need to do the job' (p. 36). Many transition from education to the workplace having had a very poor and high stress inducing experience in the education system, and this compounds the levels of anxiety that most people, even without a disability, experience when entering the world of employment for the first time. Their experience of education can induce negative expectations of the labour market and a hope that work will be different. Many hope that they will be able to leave behind the negativity of education, shutting the door on the feelings of failure and lack of ability and opening the door to a more positive environment, where people do not necessarily need to know about their condition and the likely consequences of it. A new job or workplace is always challenging for anyone, but for those with an IPD, this can also lead further to feelings of vulnerability and weakness.

Fawcett (2003) conducted an international survey of literacy which appeared to show that the levels of literacy required for employment had gone up within the last 30–40 years, making employability, for those with any form of literacy difficulties, increasingly more difficult. She predicted that this would continue to rise in the future, making it increasingly difficult to access and remain in work.

> Higher levels of literacy are demanded in employment than ever before in the history of the UK.
>
> (Fawcett, 2003, p. 99)

Such a prediction makes the process of carefully selecting a career choice increasingly important, and one that probably needs skilled and knowledgeable people to help with this. It also raises the possibility that those with an IPD make inappropriate choices of careers in the first place. Kirk and Reid (2001) showed that many selected employment that was not conducive to their particular skills, which instantly sets them up for further failure. It is possible that this is because they have not had appropriate careers advice and thereby underestimated the level of literacy required for a particular employment choice.

According to Long and Hubble (2019), in a House of Commons briefing paper, it is widely acknowledged that careers advice in schools in the UK has long been inadequate and, rather than an improving picture, there appears to be a worrying picture of deterioration of provision, both in quantity and quality, despite placing a clear duty on schools and colleges to provide impartial quality advice and expert guidance. Long and Hubble (2019) suggest that many schools and colleges need additional support to ensure that all young people, regardless of background, location, ability, race, gender and socioeconomic status, receive the appropriate advice and guidance to fulfil their potential and contribute positively to society. The DfE (2018) report on careers advice in schools reported that schools have a statutory responsibility to deliver quality careers advice and their first imperative was as follows:

> good careers guidance connects learning to the future. It motivates young people by giving them a clearer idea of the routes to jobs and careers that they will find engaging and rewarding. Good careers guidance widens pupils' horizons, challenges stereotypes and raises aspirations. It provides pupils with the knowledge and skills necessary to make successful transitions to the next stage of their life. This supports social mobility by improving opportunities for all young people, especially those from disadvantaged backgrounds and those with special educational needs and disabilities.
>
> (DfE, 2018, p. 13)

This same report describes quality careers advice as a duty for all schools, which should help pupils make an informed choice about their future lives. However, the report also recognises that on average, schools are only achieving 50% of the quality benchmarks that the government recommends, and worryingly, 20% are not hitting any of the benchmarks demanded. The State of the Nation report (Compass, 2017), proposed by Compass Careers Enterprise Company, recommended that all careers advice needed to start earlier in schools than it currently does. This would be particularly important for those with an IPD, who may find it particularly difficult to align with a particular career path and decision making. For those with an IPD it is particularly important that they are able to take a holistic view of employment, and that it is not just a subject taught as part of Personal, Social and Health Education (PSHE), but is spread across the curriculum with all teachers involved.

> This brings the subject to life and makes connections between classroom learning and young people's aspirations.
>
> (Compass, 2017, p. 28)

REFLECT ON THIS

1. Given the broad definition of dyslexia in this text, how important is it to see dyslexia as part of an IPD rather than restricting it to a literacy paradigm?
2. How could you support a work colleague, who you may suspect has an IPD, to self-disclose, and get the appropriate accommodation that they need?
3. Make a list of the challenges, as you see them, for the individual with an IPD in the workplace.
4. What cost effective accommodations could be made to overcome each of these challenges?

Interview

James is the senior manager of a medium sized manufacturing company in the North West of England; he describes a difficulty which he experienced with the workforce when trying to implement a change in systems.

> I initially wondered if the workforce were being intransigent, as it was proving very difficult to get anything implemented, the pinnacle of tenacity came when we tried to implement a system that requires operators to write things down on cards, to make the system work. Well, that was a big issue and one which the union opposed as well as the men.
>
> We struggled for around two years not realising that the reality was that 80% of the workforce had a reading and writing age below the minimum requirement of an 11-year-old.
>
> The big break came with the advent of the opening of Eastern Bloc countries, and the influx of Poles etc into the UK. Concerns over whether they could read or take oral safety instructions led us to introduce testing in maths and English. We worked with the local FE college, and together

decided that a minimum standard of capability was that of an 11-year-old, so this is where we set the test papers. In order not to be racist we implemented the test to everyone, not just those from non-British origin. The results were startling, virtually everyone from the Eastern Bloc passed, and everyone locally just about failed. Talking to the local college we found out that the area is particularly poor for numeracy and literacy with 80% of everyone in the area leaving school with a reading and writing capability either at or below that required as the minimum standard for an 11-year-old.

To begin with, we needed to get everyone over their concern about education, we couldn't just insist they had education. The first stage was to ask the college to carry out an NVQ course which was all practically based, this allowed everyone to achieve an NVQ that was equivalent to five GCSEs at grade C or above. This we did, it took six months, and everyone passed and attained their NVQ. On the back of this we introduced adult education in practical maths and English, with tutors on site from the local college. Uptake initially was poor, however through discussions with the union and making it a requirement for some disciplines, and just keeping at it, we got a significant number on the course. One other method we used was to make a selection for redundancy based on having a minimum standard for maths and English of an 11-year-old, this helped a lot!

The other change that we made was to recognise that pictures were quicker and easier to understand than text. The Track and Trace system which we introduced was both text and pictures and videos with voice-over to make sure everyone understood what was required. The T and T made reading and IT skills a real necessity and again with the college, we continue to educate the workforce. With easy steps we were able to move further forward with both more advanced machines and Track and Trace system.

In this instance James does not differentiate between those with low literacy and those with dyslexia but provided skills and training for all employees who were willing to embark on the training, making this acknowledgement of learning a positive culture within the workplace.

Going it alone

A number of researchers, including Logan (2009), have suggested that compensatory strategies that individuals with dyslexia have had to adopt to survive in education could be the very strategies that help them to enter the world of business as an employer and entrepreneur. In particular, they have often developed an advanced ability to delegate. Logan (2009) describes delegation as an *essential strength* for those who succeed in enabling their business to grow. Another compensatory strategy often used by those with an IPD is skilled oral communication; many have had to use these skills in education to overcome their lower levels of written and literacy communication. This is clearly a valuable skill for anybody setting up their own business and honing their entrepreneurial skills.

Research undertaken by Malpas (2018), and presented to the All Party Parliamentary Group (APPG) conference (APPG, 2019), showed that there were many contributors to success for those with dyslexia in employment, but interestingly education was not really one of them! Only 9% of the sample felt that their school days contributed to their employment success, whereas 72% felt that they had succeeded *because* of their dyslexia and not in spite of it, implying that there were attributes to dyslexia that were both positive and dynamic. The randomly selected sample taken by Malpas (2018), also listed these vital factors for success:

- Determination 56%
- Empathy 23%
- Intelligence or a particular ability 23%
- Motivated by helping others 19%
- Supportive family 19%
- Hard work 14%
- Effective education 9%
- Wit 6%.

It is interesting to note that a supportive family was quite high on the list and Logan (2009) also emphasised the importance of family members as mentors and role models, to encourage confidence and success in the individual with dyslexia.

REFLECT ON THIS

> The success of dyslexic people may depend on the attitudes to both their weaknesses and their experience of failure. Are the obstacles they encountered stumbling blocks or steppingstones? One of the abilities of many successful dyslexic people is to respond creatively to turn their weaknesses into strengths.
> (Morgan and Klein, 2000, p. 126)

1. Consider this quotation by Morgan and Klein (2000). How far do you think that this is true?
2. Can the experience of failure be turned into a positive?
3. What factors do you think need to be in place before a failure can be seen as a positive?
4. How can a mentor or a role model help this process?

Interview

Barry runs an engineering firm where the gender balance is almost entirely male and there are a range of nationalities. They had difficulties when asking employers and employees to undertake packing components. Many of the packages contained too many or too few of the components; it was soon realised that many of the employees were unable to successfully read the instructions they had been issued.

> Recruitment prior to 2003 was largely from recommendations by family and friends, but this was a bit incestuous. This avoided advertising and any intensive interviews however, this was not seen as satisfactory, as many were just not up to the job.
>
> Since 2003 an employment agency was recruited to manage the personnel. They advertised, interviewed and undertook all the appropriate paperwork for us.
>
> In all the years that I have been managing this factory I have never been told by any new recruit that they were dyslexic or had limited reading capabilities. I can understand why an interviewee would not want to inform their employer of this disability for fear of discrimination.

Interview

Penny is a fifty-two-year-old mother of two girls. She was born in Berlin of a British army officer and a gypsy Romany mother. She was one of seven siblings. Penny is dyslexic along with at least one of her siblings. Penny suffered considerable abuse from her father and at the age of eleven was placed in care, initially in a children's home and later with foster parents. She was moved around a lot so attended a number of different schools. However, her attendance was very limited. Her dyslexic sister was bullied in school due to her inability to read effectively and eventually gave up school. She has two daughters in their twenties, one of whom is severely dyslexic like herself, and one of her children (Penny's grandson) is also suspected of having an IPD. Her second daughter is in the police force and apparently unaffected.

Once at secondary school Penny found that it was so hard to cope as she was unable to read, having severe visual disturbances and as she describes it *the words move about the page.* When talking about her dyslexia she says that she can read the words but there is no understanding. Inevitably she became disruptive in school and the teachers did not want her in the classroom and used to tell her to: *Go outside and have a fag!* She was severely bullied in school by other children who thought she must be 'thick'. There was one teacher who she still remembers vividly, the art teacher, Penny has considerable skills in this area and considerable artistic flair. This was the only teacher who in her words, *gave her time,* and it was at this point (fourteen years of age), that she was discovered to be dyslexic. She saw no point in schooling and at the age of fifteen years she went into factory work in a chicken packing factory.

However, despite all this Penny recognised that without being able to read she was unlikely to ever get out of factory work and she did not want *to be like them.* The money she earned in the factory paid for her to have private English and maths lessons; however as much as she tried, it did not solve the issue. *I can see the words on the page, but their meaning will not go in.* She also attended free maths lessons at the local library, but these also did not help.

> I met my husband when we were children, so he knew about my difficult upbringing and after not seeing him for several years we met up again and married. I would be dead without him and his understanding of my problems. He is the only person who really knows, and I manage to cover up my problems so that no-one else is aware.

Penny went through some very difficult times, needing psychiatric help for obsessive compulsive disorder.

Penny now works with people with learning difficulties, which she feels she can empathise with. She has a responsible role, having worked her way through the system from a volunteer (so has never had to complete a CV), but her employers are unaware that she has low literacy. She attends meetings and often is required to deliver presentations to the team. The way that she deals with this is to take all the minutes home with her, learn things by heart, and her daughter reads the material to her, taping it to her phone. Between her daughter and her husband, she prepares all written material at home before attending meetings. Penny is very talented in art and prepares large pictorial mind maps to share with the team. These mind maps are also what she uses with the people that she works with, who find them invaluable to their learning. All Penny's teaching is based on these mind maps.

When asked to talk about her dyslexia her response was:

> Oh my God I hate it! I hate not being able to do it [read] it is so embarrassing. I am so ashamed, and I hate having to ask for help from my daughter and husband. It is not even big words that are a problem, sometimes it is simple words like 'the'. I have to do a lot of pretending and a lot of sweating when I do not understand. I hate it, I hate it, I hate it. I feel so thick.

I know that it was very hard for Penny to give me this interview and talk about such difficult periods in her life, and I am so grateful that she felt able to be so open and honest with me.

Chapter reflections

The Basic Skills Agency completed a survey in 1997, which estimated that the cost related to employment of low literacy was approximately £4.8 billion per annum; that included lost tax revenue, lost national insurance, unemployment and other state benefits. With a disputed estimate of inflation at 2.78% per annum over the last twenty-two years, this adds up to a colossal sum of money which, if even a tiny fraction were reallocated to improving literacy in this country, could be an immense benefit to society and to the lives of the many individuals. This chapter has shown that far more work needs to be done to establish quality careers advice for young people with IPDs and also to raise awareness among employers and human resource departments to understand the needs of those with an IPD and also to understand the considerable benefits that employing these people can bring to their companies.

This theme will be continued in the next chapter which will take this concept even further and suggest that far from being a drain on society, those who think differently can positively contribute to the world's economy by recognising and using the considerable strengths and talents that many with IPDs appear to have.

Further reading

Hagan, B (2014) *Dyslexia in the Workplace: A TUC Guide* (3rd edn). www.tuc.org.uk (accessed 02.12.19).

This is a leaflet filled with useful and practical information for any employer or employee. It is written by Brian Hagan, who has been a committed TUC member for over thirty-eight years, but importantly Hagan is also a teacher of adults with dyslexia, and his passion for this comes through in his writing. His particular interest is in ensuring that reasonable adjustments are identified for each individual, and then implemented in the workplace when they are needed. He explains in readable terms the implications of the Equality Act 2010 to both employees and employers. He emphasises the need for a proactive approach to dyslexia and employment, whilst also recognising the challenges within a difficult labour market.

This is a short and very accessible guide and should be essential reading for all workplace managers of both small and large organisations.

References

All Party Parliamentary Group for Dyslexia and other SpLDs (APPG) (2019) *The Human Cost of Dyslexia: The Emotional and Psychological Impact of Poorly Supported Dyslexia.* BDA. www.bdadyslexia.org.uk/about/all-party-parliamentary-group-dyslexia-and-spld-appg (accessed 01. 12. 19).

Basic Skills Agency (1997) *Staying the Course: The Relationship Between Basic Skills Support, Drop Out, Retention and Achievement in Further Education Colleges.* London: Basic Skills Agency.

Beetham, J (2018) Employers: making reasonable adjustments. In *The Dyslexia Handbook 2018.* Bracknell: BDA.

British Dyslexia Association (2019) *Dyslexia.* www.bdadyslexia.org.uk/dyslexia (accessed 01. 12. 19).

Compass (2017) *State of the Nation 2017: Careers and Enterprise Provision in England's Schools.* London: The Careers and Enterprise Company.

Dale, C and Aiken, F (2007) *A Review of the Literature into Dyslexia in Nursing Practice.* Royal College of Nursing. http://www.uhs.nhs.uk/Media/suhtideal/NursesAndMidwives/PreQualifyingNursing/RCNreportdyslexiaandpractice.pdf (accessed 04. 12. 19).

Department for Education (DfE) (2018), *Careers Guidance and Access for Education and Training Providers Statutory Guidance for Governing Bodies, School Leaders and School Staff.* London: Crown.

Department of Health (DoH) (2019) *Advice for Employers on Workplace Adjustments for Mental Health Conditions.* www.centreformentalhealth.org.uk/sites/default/files/mental_health_adjustments_guidance_may_2012_dh.pdf (accessed 01. 12. 19).

Eide, BL and Eide, FF (2011) *The Dyslexic Advantage: Unlocking the Hidden Potential of the Dyslexic Brain.* London: Hey House UK Ltd.

Equality Act (2010) www.legislation.gov.uk/ukpga/2010/15/contentsLondon: HMSO (accessed 02. 12. 19).

Equality and Human Rights Commission (2016) *In Employment: Workplace Adjustments.* www.equalityhumanrights.com/en (accessed 02. 12. 19).

Fitzgibbon, G and O'Connor, B (2002) *Adult Dyslexia: A guide for the workplace.* Chichester: John Wiley and Sons Ltd.

Fawcett, A (2003) *Dyslexia: A Psychological Perspective.* Oxford: Blackwell Publishing.

Gibb, N (2015) Address to the Education Reform Summit. www.gov.uk/government/speeches/the-purpose-of-education (accessed 20. 06. 19).

Hagan, B (2014) *Dyslexia in the Workplace: A TUC Guide* (3rd edn). www.tuc.org.uk (accessed 02. 12. 19).

Hoffmann, FJ, Sheldon, KL, Minskoff, EH, Sauter, SW, Steidle, EF, Baker, DP, Bailey, MB and Echols, LD (1987) Needs of learning disabled adults. *Journal of Learning Disabilities* 20(1): 43–52.

Kirk, J and Reid, G (2001) An examination of the relationship between dyslexia and offending in young people and the implications for the training system. *Dyslexia* 7(2): 77–84.

Logan, J (2009) *Dyslexic Entrepreneurs: The Incidence; Their Coping Strategies and Their Business Skills.* London: Dyslexia. www.interscience.wiley.com (accessed 02. 12. 19).

Long R and Hubble S (2019) *Careers Guidance in Schools, Colleges and Universities.* House of Commons briefing paper, Number 07236, 23 April 2019, House of Commons Library Research Service.

Malpas, M (2018) *Under Your Nose: How to release talent from your neuro-diverse workforce.* Presentation to the APPG19 November 2018. www.bdadyslexia.org.uk/about/all-party-parliamentary-group-dyslexia-and-spld-appg (accessed 01. 12. 19).

Morgan, E and Klein, C (2000) *The Dyslexic Adult: In a Non-dyslexic World.* London: Whurr.

Scott, R (2004) *Dyslexia and Counselling.* London: Whurr Publishers Ltd.

Shakespeare, W (reproduced 1978) *The Complete Works of Shakespeare.* Hamlet: Prince of Denmark. London: Abbey Library.

Vogel, SA and Adelman, PB (2000) Adults with learning disabilities 8–15 years after college. *Learning Disabilities: A Multi-disciplinary Journal* 10(3): 165–182.

8 Balancing the books
Advantages to society

Introduction

The content and tone of this chapter will be very different to the rest of the book, as instead of focussing upon the challenges and difficulties for those with an information processing difference (IPD), this chapter will be one of celebration and positivity. The chapter will examine how *because* of their dyslexia, and not in spite of it, those with these conditions can succeed, as they draw on their strengths and talents to reap the benefits of the different ways in which their brain works. This chapter aims to redress the balance and enable you to understand how by nurturing these talents those who think differently can contribute positively to the economy, and can create a return on investment that far outweighs the costs and interventions of support and remediation.

To this point the book has concentrated upon the negative side of IPDs, of poverty, mental health issues, unemployment, etc.; however, there is a more positive side to the dyslexia coin, and it can be viewed in a different way, opposite but the same. Every day has a night and without the dark you cannot appreciate the light, but sometimes the dark drowns out the light, and you need to step back to see the positive side shining through. Chapter five in this book showed how education and teaching in this country is so heavily focused upon reading and literacy that those with any form of IPD will probably find formal education very hard. However, with the arrival of adulthood, people can be free from the areas that they find so challenging, and can use the talents and skills that their particular brain structure lends itself to, and can blossom into innovative, creative and unique individuals.

Strengths can overcome weaknesses

There is no doubt that in education, and in particular in schools, having an IPD is difficult, and is described by the government as a disability (DfE/DoH 2015), that is, you have a long-term physical or mental impairment. This is only because the things that society values, at this period in our evolution, are heavily reliant upon reading, writing, spelling, short-term memory, processing speed and language development, and all the support and guidance at this time is focused upon improving reading and literacy. It is a bit like walking down a long dark tunnel, because there is a tiny glimpse of light at the end, but ignoring the many escape hatches along the way that could lead the individual into the light open spaces that allow them to flower in a different way. The escape hatches could allow the person with an IPD to escape from the confines of the tunnel that everyone else travels along and thereby achieve the freedom to develop alternative talents.

Eide and Eide (2011) emphasise the need to see those with IPDs as a two-sided, neurological coin: on the one side are the great challenges that are commonly associated with these conditions and on the other side are the strengths that are just as much a part of the condition as the challenges, but are not so often acknowledged. There is no such thing as a one-sided coin, and whatever we see on the one side, when we turn it over there will always be something else, possibly brighter and shinier, on the other.

> Strengths are as much a part of the dyslexic profile as challenges in reading and spelling.
>
> (Eide and Eide, 2011, p. 17)

However, it is not possible, under current research ethics, to say whether these strengths have occurred as a direct result of this brain difference, or as a secondary, more environmentally attributable result. An example of this could be that experiencing constant failure in school and education could potentially produce a more resilient individual with greater determination to succeed.

Eide and Eide (2011) developed the acronym MIND strengths, whilst not denying the challenges for those with dyslexia they also observed, in their research, many strengths and they listed these as creative qualities.

M – *Material reasoning*. This, according to Eide and Eide (2011), is the ability to 'see' objects in space, with a heightened awareness of shape, size and position, in 3D. They recognised that this ability was not an area highly prized within the school curriculum, but that it is phenomenally useful to many occupations, such as designers, engineers, skilled artisans, architects, scientists, etc. The M strengths require an advanced ability to imagine a shape in space and time, and an ability to manipulate that shape by rotation, repositioning and interconnectivity.

I – *Interconnected reasoning*. This is the ability to identify patterns and relationships by noticing similarities and differences, and to bring these different parts together to perceive a whole, whilst understanding its core meaning.

On a hot sunny day my severely dyslexic six-year-old son and I were lying on the grass looking up at the clouds. I could see clouds! He could see castles and dragons and whole stories scudding through the sky, with one idea leading to another.

N – *Narrative reasoning*. This is the ability to use past, personal experience and memories to put new situations into context. This ability to see a mental scenario is a highly creative form of thinking. This is the capacity to weave narrative stories and it is common to many high-profile and published writers who have declared their dyslexia, such as Lynda La Plante (author of the books and TV series *Prime Suspect*), Richard Ford (author of *Sportswriter*), John Irving (*The Cider House Rules*), F. Scott Fitzgerald (of *Great Gatsby* fame) etc. All these writers demonstrate a remarkable capacity to write with such richness of detail, extraordinary plot lines, observational analogy and imagery.

D – *Dynamic reasoning*. This is the ability to predict what might happen in relation to past experiences, and to create working hypotheses for situations which have not yet happened or are not yet possible. These are the problem solvers of this world, able to see change, uncertainty and ambiguity and yet to work with this to a more positive outcome. This level of dynamic reasoning and insightfulness can be seen in entrepreneurs, for example, Sir Richard Branson (founder of Virgin), Ingvar Kmprad (founder of IKEA), Dame Anita Roddick (founder of Bodyshop), Paul Orfale (founder of Kinkos), etc., all of whom are self-declared dyslexics. What all of these have in common is a level of optimism and resilience, the ability to recognise their personal strengths and reframe their challenges and setbacks into positive experiences. If accurately calculated Virgin Business Enterprises, founded by Sir Richard Branson, on its own had a net worth of £17.5 billion in 2019, so the net worth to the British economy of just one of these entrepreneurs is immense (Companies House, 2019).

Stereotypes and Savant Syndrome

The strengths of dyslexia are the same as the definition for dyslexia itself; like shifting sand and difficult to pin down, every study appears to have their own contenders. Claims for such strengths are many and various, but the problem appears to be that whilst these characteristics are frequently seen in an individual with dyslexia, they are not seen in *every* individual with dyslexia. In the same way as films such as the 1988 *Rain Man*, starring Dustin Hoffman, popularised the stereotype that all individuals with autism have high functioning abilities, the truth is probably that whilst *some* do, many do not. This is not very helpful to those who want to study the characteristics of dyslexia and IPDs. In Table 8.1, I have pulled together what I will call *representative strengths*, from other researchers in this field, to compile a quite extensive list; once again it is important to emphasise that not all those with dyslexia will have all or even any of these.

Scott (2004) even goes as far as to say that dyslexia as a strength is important for the survival of the human species, and believes that over the millennia it has been a species advantage which has help humans to emerge as the most resourceful of the animal kingdom. Literacy is a recent cultural invention, rather than an adaptation of natural selection, and at a time when reading and literacy were unknown and not relevant to survival, to have an individual with these exceptional talents of creativity and intuitive thinking within a group could, quite literally, have been the difference between life and death.

Table 8.1 Some of the talents attributed to dyslexia

High levels of creativity.	Outstanding visual/spatial skills, so good at solving puzzles and breaking codes.	Good declarative learning (learning facts – all dogs are canines – rather than knowing how to do something – drive a car).
Good semantic memory. That is, knowing facts such as colours or dog breeds as opposed to episodic memory – what happened last night.	Good social skills.	High levels of resilience and perseverance, concentration and persistence.
Intuitive and insightful thinking.	Multi-dimensional thought and pictorial thinkers.	Focused.
Rapid grasp of new concepts.	Awareness of patterns, connections and relationships in diverse perspectives.	Energy levels high.
High levels of curiosity.	Self-aware.	Proactive.
Good at goal setting.	Good at design development.	Empathetic.
Able to communicate ideas.	Vivid imagination.	Able to motivate and lead.
Able to delegate.	Abstract thinkers, using pictures to think.	Finds alternative and innovative uses for objects.
A holistic thinker, able to see the big picture without getting lost in the detail.	Good reasoning skills.	Heightened peripheral vision.
Excellent problem solvers with innovative styles of thinking.	Creative and original.	Entrepreneurial.

It is not a mistake, it is not an accident. It is not a human trait that is suited to a literate society, but, for it to have remained in our genetic inheritance, there must be some importance to dyslexia for human survival.

(Scott, 2004, pp. 10–11)

A very rare condition, usually associated with autism and other IPDs, is Savant Syndrome (the literal meaning of savant is scholar). This is a condition whereby despite being significantly disabled by their condition, the individual also has outstanding skills, usually associated with areas of memory, such as maths, music, art, spatial location ability (maps), perfect appreciation of the passing of time (without using a clock or watch), the capacity to measure distances without instruments or occasionally advanced verbal skills and foreign language learning. This may also manifest itself in an obsessive preoccupation with a particular thing, such as car licence plate numbers, train numbers and identification. It is important to understand that savants are not geniuses and it can occur within the full range of IQ scores, but they have one or more exceptional talents, usually related to memory. An example of a dyslexic savant can be seen in the Hindi film *Taare Zameen Par* (2007) (*Stars upon the Ground*), which portrays an eight-year-old boy who is severely tormented at school for being dyslexic and unable to read or write, until his art teacher takes a particular interest in this little boy, and reveals his amazing artistic talents. This is a classic portrayal of a dyslexic savant.

Savant Syndrome truly is a juxtaposition of ability and disability in the one individual, and an extreme example of the remarkable plasticity of the brain, which Treffert (2014) called 'islands of genius'.

> Extraordinary strengths are the exception rather than the rule even in dyslexia, but strengths in dyslexia tend to emerge after the school years. These 'learned talents' may keep developing, often through the variety of experiences gained.
>
> (Nicholson, 2015, p. 42)

It is highly likely, although very difficult to prove, that creative individuals such as Leonardo da Vinci and Albert Einstein were dyslexic savants, as both are recorded as having difficulties with reading and spelling despite their amazing achievements in art and science.

Entrepreneurs and employment

According to the Forbes World Billionaires list (2019), Sir Richard Branson, founder of the Virgin Group, probably has a personal fortune of approximately 4.1 billion pounds, Sir Alan Sugar, the property tycoon and star of the TV programme *The Apprentice*, is probably worth 1.2 billion pounds and Donald Trump, president of America and businessman, probably 3.5 billion dollars. What these all have in common is that they are entrepreneurs and they all have self-declared dyslexia. These are only a few of the many successful entrepreneurs who are dyslexic or have IPDs. Research by Logan (2010) showed that the number of entrepreneurs with dyslexia in the UK is approximately 19% and the number in the USA is even higher at over 30%; both these figures far exceed the estimated number of people with dyslexia in the population as a whole. It is interesting that in Logan's research, this figure is not replicated in the number of corporate managers which is nearer to 1% and 3% respectively. Logan (2010) suggests that the reason for this is that as an entrepreneur, individuals have more control over their environment, which better suits the information processing style and right brained thinking of those with dyslexia. Logan (2010) surmises that because of their poor reading and writing skills the individual with dyslexia will try to compensate by developing excellent communication skills and can therefore develop close and dynamic teams around them.

The difficulties that are experienced by those with dyslexia are largely due to living in a society that values literacy so highly and perhaps, as we move forward with technology, this will not always be the case, and the strengths that have helped these entrepreneurs to succeed will become more relevant to employment in a less reading based culture. Perhaps we are already seeing a change in the world of work as employment relies more on computers and technology, digitalisation, artificial intelligence, 3D printing and biotechnology. The organisation Made by Dyslexia (2018) believes that this could be shifting the balance to the need for more creative and innovative thinkers with the flexibility to adapt quickly to a fast-paced world. This could present a potential skills gap, and one that many with IPDs are ideally placed to fill. It is likely that currently we have a large pool of, as yet undervalued, talent which could become the *most wanted* employees of the future, who could drive society forward and even get us out of the overwhelmingly frightening climate change and enviro-terrorism problems that we appear to have created for ourselves ... literally saving the planet! For this to happen employers, governments, corporations and the world of work worldwide need to have a much more proactive and high-profile neuro-diverse strategy for recruitment, with the ability to accurately map intuitive abilities to the needs of their companies and countries, not only now, but into the foreseeable future.

> In many industries and countries, the most in-demand occupations or specialities did not exist 10 or even five years ago, and the pace of change is set to accelerate. By one particular estimate, 65% of children entering primary school today will ultimately end up working in completely new jobs, types that don't yet exist.
>
> (World Economic Forum, 2016, p. 3)

The World Economic Forum (2016), calls this the Fourth Industrial Revolution. This same report calculates that from 2020, a third of all jobs will need employees who have complex problem-solving skills, and this will be overwhelmingly the most sort-after ability of the future, closely followed by social skills, coincidentally the two skills that many of those with IPDs are reported to excel at. For those with an IPD it is important to remember what Nicolson (2015) puts so well:

> No-one will ever employ you because your reading has got less bad – they will employ you because of your strengths.
>
> (Nicolson, 2015: p. 1)

Mentors and friends

In Rooke's (2016) book about successful dyslexics, twenty-three famous and celebrated people with dyslexia talk honestly about their experience of living with the condition, and the positive impact they believe it had on their lives and their ability to succeed. The contributors range from TV broadcasters, sports personalities, dancers, poets and authors. The one thing that they all seem to have in common is self-belief and a determination to overcome the challenges that they face. Reading each vignette, it is interesting to see how many times they attribute that self-belief to one person in their lives who could see their potential, despite their difficulties, and helped them to understand their strengths. This one person was often a family member, but just as often it was a chance encounter with a teacher, sports coach, trusted friend, work colleague, youth worker, etc. These people, often unbeknown to them, became a mentor, a person who helps another to develop themselves. These encounters are often chance affairs and could be quite brief or long-lasting relationships, but all are based on trust,

An unofficial mentor, or special life person, is someone who is *just there*; they do not force their ideas on another, but are often at their most effective when they step back and allow the mentee to learn for themselves. The person with an IPD does not need someone giving out wise advice, but does need supporting behaviour, someone to recognise when they do well: this is what could be described as enabling self-sufficiency. This special person in the life of the individual with dyslexia is often completely unaware of the impact they are having, simply by being there and providing a sounding board, allowing *safe* opportunities for the mentee to let off steam. They are frequently referred to as an inspiration and someone who *opened doors* to the future.

We have probably all had an unofficial mentor at some point in our lives (initially they are probably a parent), but it is someone who is interested in us and we instinctively turn to when support and guidance is needed. This is really about a relationship rather than a function and may not even be recognised as mentoring. It may not even be intentional, and it just emerges with someone who helped us through problems, allowed us to grow and develop, but most importantly allowed us to feel good about ourselves by helping us to find our own answers. For someone with an IPD it is imperative that this unofficial mentor is able to recognise their abilities through mutual respect, and makes it clear, by their actions, that they believe in them and their capacity to achieve, like a nurturing and reassuring parental figure.

Brain structure

A full scientific understanding of dyslexia and IPDs is still some way off, but an examination of post mortem brains and the use of functional magnetic resonance images (fMRI) does appear to show some anatomical variations, particularly in the left hemisphere, known to be responsible for phonological processing, fine detail processing and working memory (Figure 8.1). Wolf (2008) indicates that the right side of the brain, or right hemisphere, is responsible for 'big picture' thinking and at making connections and finding relationships between ideas. These ideas can then be manipulated in the right hemisphere to perceive a global understanding of all the component parts. Eide and Eide (2011) use the analogy of being able to link the component parts of eyes, nose and mouth into the image of a whole distinguishable face another example would be to understand how individual leaves, twigs and branches build into a whole tree and eventually a forest. An extensive review of the available in vivo research studies by Sun et al. (2010) disclosed that many showed significant differences between the brains of those who were neuro-diverse and those who were neuro-typical, in particular, differences in the ratio of grey matter to white matter and in the symmetry of the two hemispheres, producing a different pattern of communication between the two hemispheres. Studies using magnetic resonance imaging (MRI), functional magnetic resonance imaging (fMRI), magnetic resonance spectroscopy (MRS), diffusion tensor imaging (DTI), positron emission tomography (PET), electroencephalography (EEG) and magnetoencephalography (MEG) (see glossary) were all reviewed from across the world of phonographic systems of reading and writing and most indicated either a larger right hemisphere compared to the left (in individuals without dyslexia it would be expected to see a larger left hemisphere), or a more symmetrical appearance particularly in the cerebellum (Figure 8.2). Other differences seen in the review by Sun et al. (2010) were reduced neural activity in the left temporal and left parietal cortices, and widespread activation in the cerebellum. These studies almost all indicated that those with dyslexia are right brained thinkers; in other words when they interpret the world around them, they use the right hemisphere of the brain far more than those who are not dyslexic. Sun et al. (2010) also reviewed a small number of biochemical studies, which appeared to indicate differences in the biochemical make-up of the brains in dyslexic and non-dyslexic people. The review, although comprehensive, does acknowledge that there are some variations in the results of the studies reviewed, and this is probably due to differences in scanning techniques and differences of the definition of dyslexia used, which could result in differences of the inclusion of particular participants to the studies.

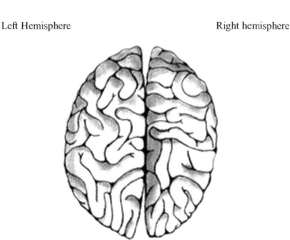

Figure 8.1 Hemispheres of the brain (diagram first published in Hayes, 2019)

134 *Balancing the books*

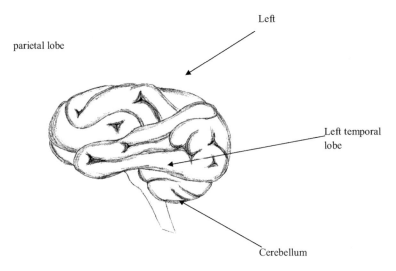

Figure 8.2 Brain structure (diagram first published in Hayes, 2019)

Eide and Eide (2011), whilst not contesting that the brain of the individual with dyslexia operates differently to the neuro-typical individual, do describe the learning process that the brain undertakes as being neither left or right brained, but rather a continuous process, combining the two hemispheres, each reliant upon the other. They suggest that when an inexperienced learner (usually a child, but not necessarily) starts to learn something new, the big picture thinking of the right hemisphere is invaluable, as it allows the new learner to see the whole new task: seeing the tree but not necessarily taking notice of the leaves and branches, seeing the essence of the task but not the nuance. This allows the brain to recognise similarities and connections to existing knowledge and understanding, allowing the new task to be chained and linked to other already established information, and to use that existing knowledge to better interpret the new.

> In these ways, the right hemisphere's top-down or big picture processing is ideal for our early attempts to stumble through processes we're still fuzzy on. It's also invaluable when we try to tackle other tasks which we lack the automatic skills to perform quickly and efficiently.
>
> (Eide and Eide, 2011, p. 34)

Eventually the brain needs to process this information from the right hemisphere to the left hemisphere, as it needs to dig deep into the fine detail, of seeing that the tree is made up of smaller and smaller individual parts, branches, twigs, leaves, veins, cells, different colours, shapes, sizes, etc. The suggestion by Eide and Eide (2011) is that perhaps this is where the processing difficulty in those with dyslexia is founded and the brain gets 'stuck' in a beginner learner mode, finding it hard to shift to towards the left hemisphere.

> dyslexic brains function differently from nondyslexic ones not because they're defective but because they're organised to display different kinds of strengths. These strengths are achieved at the cost of relative weakness in certain kinds of fine detail processing.
>
> (Eide and Eide, 2011, p. 43)

Jung-Beeman (2005) also concluded that whilst the left hemisphere was vital for comprehending language and eventually reading, the right hemisphere also has a vital role with evidence from neuropsychology, neuroimaging and neuroanatomy indicating a highly complex interaction for semantic processing.

An influential study by Williams and Casanova (2010) appeared to show what they called mini-columns of cells in the cortex of the brain. These microscopic cells seemed to be arranged vertically into tiny columns. The columns are connected by long hair-like structures called axons, linking neurons from one column to another, to form circuits. Williams and Casanova (2010) appeared to show that across a population, there was likely to be a normal distribution bell curve of those with long projections and larger spaces between mini-columns, and those with closely packed mini-columns but those at the extremes of the bell curve could be identified as dyslexia or autism, on the autistic spectrum (Figure 8.3).

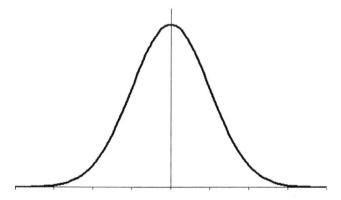

Figure 8.3 Normal distribution curve for axons

They implied that those with the longer spaced connections were better at the big picture thinking, whereas those with the closer connections were better at fine detail and component features of a task. This is, of course, a greatly simplified account of the very complex structure, anatomy and working of the brain, but does throw up some interesting areas for argument and hopefully for further future research.

REFLECT ON THIS

With a colleague or your tutor reflect on the following questions:

1 What ethical implications are there for studies such as those discussed above?
2 How can researchers maintain objectivity and ensure that both strengths and weaknesses are highlighted?
3 What special precautions do you think need to be taken when researching groups of vulnerable people, such as those with IPDs?

Big picture thinkers

Big picture thinking is something that is commonly thought to be a strength of people who are neuro-diverse and describes the ability to 'see' a whole scene to describe an incident. There is an old adage which says that a 'picture paints a thousand words', and in the case of those who are able to do this it really is true. Imagine trying to describe to someone the Mona Lisa … it could take hours, days or even weeks to fully describe what you see, books and books have been written about this most famous painting. When looking at that painting, so many thoughts and ideas flash through your brain within milliseconds, all helping to bring focus, shape, opinion and challenge to the understanding. Davis (1997) claims that picture thinking is probably between 400 and 4,000 times faster than verbal thinking. Davis (1997) also describes verbal thinking as linear and sequential, letters making words, words making sentences, sentences making paragraphs, etc. Picture thinking, however, sparks and flashes about in the brain, encompassing mental images in a very short period of time. If you close your eyes and think of a dog you probably see a whole dog, probably in context, a Labrador or a Chihuahua, on a lead, in a field, etc.; it is less likely that you will see a linear view of the scene … the tail, the hindquarters, the haunches and finally the head, before you realise that what you are seeing is a dog.

For such pictorial thinking to happen Davis (1997) believes that conscious awareness is vital for understanding. For anyone to be aware of a particular stimulus, such as a picture, it needs to be visually present for at least 1/25 of a second before it enters an individual's consciousness; this is approximately the same speed as individual film frames appear on the screen to give the impression of smooth motion. If a picture is presented at 1/36 of a second or slightly less, for example, it is unlikely that the average person would be consciously aware of it but it could arguably become subliminal, that is, perceived by the brain but the person has no awareness of it, what could be called a 'concealed memory'. Any faster than 1/36 of a second is probably too fast for the brain to register at all.

> Picture thinking seems to be consistently happening at about thirty-two pictures per second, or a frequency of 1/32 of a second, the same speed as the flicker-fusion rate of the eye.
>
> (Davis, 1997, p. 102)

Dyslexia is certainly generally perceived as a disability, and is even classified as a disability by the government (DfE/DoH, 2015), enabling those with the condition to obtain additional funding in education and reasonable adjustment in employment. It would be disingenuous to say that it does not bring with it a multitude of challenges however; the indicators of dyslexia vary widely from one individual to another, and the disadvantages do also come with some positives, which in evolutionary terms would probably have been highly beneficial. Unfortunately, what we do not yet know is whether these advantageous skills are something inherent, something about the brains of those with dyslexia and IPDs, or whether it is in some way a form of compensation for the difficulties, for example, people with dyslexia tend to read less, so there is less activity in this area of the brain. It could be that it is the constant need to challenge those difficulties and overcome the problems in neuro-diverse individuals that shapes the brain differently to the neuro-typical brain, and it is this that results in the apparent advantages of the big picture thinkers, the creative, innovative and curious brain.

Research by Schneps (2015) showed that the very act of reading can change the brain. This research appears to show that someone who reads for an hour or more a day over many years (not difficult to do when you include reading from a screen, reading posters on the train, food labels in the supermarket, reports and instructions for work and books, etc.) gives the brain *specialist repetitive training* which even makes the brain look different in scans. It must be remembered that reading requires split second eye control and information processing, and it is this that Schneps (2015) claims shapes the neural pathways in the brain to go along narrow alleyways, allowing the reader to focus on the detail required for the skill of reading. Poorer readers find this attentive focus difficult, and this could account for a learned rather than innate ability to become more globally aware and big picture thinkers (Figure 8.4).

Interview

Mustav is fifty-five years old and has his own landscape gardening business, employing twenty-five people. Mustav has been identified with dyslexia.

138 Balancing the books

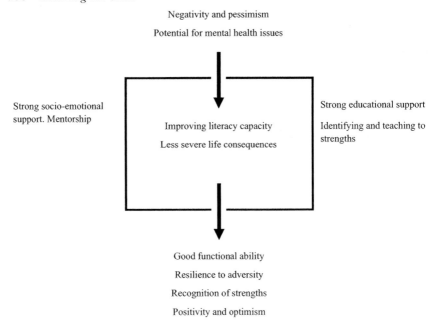

Figure 8.4 Dyslexia support

Much to my parent's disappointment I never really excelled at school, I was a diligent child and largely I managed to stay out of trouble, but never really achieved very much, as my teachers constantly told me. I hated school, I felt a failure because either explicitly or in underlying tones I was told that I was a failure. At home my grandad had an allotment which I loved to help him with. I think that I just really wanted to be with him as he was such a kind man and never made me feel that I was letting him down. I would sneak down to the allotment on my way home from school and just by being there, on my own with the plants, the smell of the soil, the tools in the shed and the huge stack of plant catalogues, which I loved to look through, seemed to wipe away all the frustrations and turmoil of the day in school.

I left school as soon as I could, my parents wanted me to stay there, like my sister, but I could not see the point. They said that I could only leave if I had a job to go to, but no one was going to employ me without qualifications. Eventually a friend of my grandad offered me a job in his horticultural business, just cutting lawns in big houses and weeding bedding areas. It was hard work and long hours, but I loved the solitude and gradually I began to feel that I had worth, I loved the power to be able to plant a seed and see it grow into such a beautiful form. Eventually I started to read about the plants that I grew and to realise the need to understand about the growing process.

I am now fifty-five years old and I am so proud of my landscape gardening business, employing twenty-five people. I have my own house with a beautiful garden. People seem to like the creative garden designs that I envision and want me to design for them. I now know that I am dyslexic and that diagnosis came as a great relief to me and only came about when I saw my grandson struggling at school in the same way that I had, and I was determined that he would not suffer in the same way as I did. When I recruit new personnel, I like to encourage others with dyslexia, as they seem to have a sixth sense for what will work in a garden. They need to understand how to 'paint' the colours on the soil with creative and innovative designs.

REFLECT ON THIS

It is said that GCHQ (Government Communications Headquarters), the intelligence gathering and security organisation, employs more than one hundred people with an IPD, (to combat terrorism and espionage); they really seem to value their amazing ability to analyse complex information skilfully and compile and decipher codes. This can be seen in their 'You See Things Differently: so we can flourish' recruitment campaign (Intelligence and Security Committee of Parliament, 2018). Employing dyslexic cryptographists can make a vital contribution to the security of this country.

1 Can you think of any other areas of employment where such neurodiverse skills could be seen to be an advantage?
2 How could the identification of dyslexia in adults become a positive catalyst for change?

Creativity and curiosity

Creativity is intuitive, it is inventive, and it is what has allowed humans to move out of the caves, discover fire, develop machines and learn ever new ways to preserve and extend life. Creativity is about original thinking, and some people with IPDs do seem to have that ability to think outside the box and to be resourceful enough to come up with original and inventive ideas to solve problems. Creativity allows humans to reason and use logic and to use experimentation to produce inventive solutions to problems, making this ability both useful to mankind in general, but also productive and economically successful.

Cancer et al. (2016) conducted a small-scale piece of research to examine whether there was a significant link between those with identified dyslexia and creativity. The results of their research did appear to show that in *some* individuals there was a high correlation between certain types of creative thinking and dyslexia; however, this has not always been found and a case study by Mourgues et al. (2014) showed less conclusive results. Anecdotally however,

140 *Balancing the books*

these high levels of creativity do appear to be recognised as a strength of dyslexia, so much so that in America some firms that value inventive intuition, such as architects, actively encourage applications from individuals with dyslexia, and even in the UK there are employment agencies specifically finding jobs for those they describe as *exceptional people*.

Redefining success

Success is just another concept that you have encountered in this book that is difficult to define. Success means different things to different people: to some it may be related to employment, or physical prowess on a racetrack or a sports field, to some it will mean family success, building relationships, etc. Typically, success is measured in terms of material wealth, who has the bigger, faster car or better more palatial house; money is a key indicator of success with status and influence also high in the success stakes of society, but happiness or emotional success is also important. This really all depends upon what we value as a society and as an individual, but equally what society values is often valued by the individual (Figure 8.5).

Redefining what we see as success probably means a more sophisticated idea of what contributes to success, to those with IPDs success can probably be measured by the ability to be fully literate, but this is too narrow and based against very subjective criteria. Unless society and employers are able to make systematic changes, then inclusion and equality cannot be achieved, celebrating the diversity of talent. A definition of success needs to be diverse, based on how an individual feels about themselves and what they see as the achievements that really matter to them. This level of diversity really matters to society, if we were all successful at the same thing (which is frequently seen in education, where success is measured in everyone achieving the same high grades in the same subject areas), then society would grind to a halt. We need people to be successful at a complete range of skills, knowledge and understanding, leading teams, running the library, coaching the sports people, medicine, accounting, gardening, building, driving, making things etc.

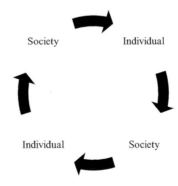

Figure 8.5 Redefining success

Interview

Chung-ho was born in this country of Asian parents. He now runs a very successful restaurant specialising in a range of Asian foods; he is about to open another restaurant and is looking for a chef to run the kitchen, but he is keen to find and help someone who has dyslexia and is as passionate about food as he is.

> I really struggled at school, I spoke the language of my family at home, but always remember speaking English, and would see English as my first language. I really struggled at school and teachers seemed to believe that it was because of the bilingualism but I just knew that this was not the problem. I was always slower than everyone in my class to produce work and always got the lowest marks. I just did not seem to be able to find any subject that I could excel in ... school was a very miserable time for me and I don't mind telling you, that in my teens I even considered suicide, as life just did not seem worth living. This was a very dark period of my life, as my parents could only see success at school as the way forward for me and I know that they were very worried about what would happen to me.
>
> I used to help my mum in the kitchen and used to love to watch her making some wonderful dishes, that we all enjoyed. She was so creative and was keen to mix and match flavours, she just seemed to know what would work well together, even when it was unusual. However, she kept shooing me out of the kitchen, saying that I needed to do my homework.
>
> When I was fifteen, I just knew that I could not stay in school any more and against my parents' wishes I left and got a job helping in the kitchen of the local restaurant. This was an epiphany ... suddenly I realised what I really wanted to do. The chef was wonderful and realised that I had potential and he nurtured me and encouraged me to go to college to do a catering course. Somehow the struggle with reading did not seem so great when I was reading and writing about something that I was passionate about. This was the outlet for my creativity and flair that I needed, and I have now won several awards for my innovative and imaginative recipes. The first time I won an award my mum was so proud of me she told all the neighbours about her son who had won an award!

Chapter reflections

Going forward employers need to look again at the neurodiversity of their workforce and consider how the strengths shown by those with IPDs can be used to benefit their companies. They need to train their senior staff and recruitment officers to spot these talents at interview, even in those who present with less than conventional qualifications and experience, by advanced skills mapping. The false perception of dyslexia as a negative must be mitigated, and a more positive view of the condition adopted, putting forward a strengths based approach to education and employment and redefining the meaning of success.

Despite the strengths that have been outlined in this chapter, there has to be some sense of realism as well; dyslexia will always present immense challenges to individuals struggling to cope in a *reading society*. The general public, many of whom will be bosses and recruitment agents, currently frequently see dyslexia as a substantial disability, believing that it means that the individual with dyslexia is illiterate and thereby a risk to employment, but just because there may be difficulties in one area of learning this should not prevent success in other areas. This chapter shows that not every individual with IPDs will have extraordinary talents, but each will be a unique individual with often unrealized potential and worthy of supporting to bring that potential to the forefront of their employment. Convincing individuals with dyslexia of their strengths is hard enough, but perhaps the bigger challenge is to convince wider society of the advantages of dyslexia to their businesses, to society and to the economy.

> The key point is that these weaknesses reflect learning differences, not learning disabilities. For every downside, there is an upside, and the key plan is to work smarter, being aware of and tolerant to your weaknesses, so that you can transform them into distinctive strengths, A weakness is a half-way house to a strength.
>
> (Nicolson, 2015, p. 118)

Further reading

Eide, BL and Eide, FF (2011) *The Dyslexia Advantage: Unlocking the Hidden Potential of the Dyslexic Brain*. London: Hay House UK Ltd.

This book attempts to shift thinking about dyslexia from the negative to the positive, to encourage professionals and lay people alike that for people with dyslexia there is a light at the end of the educational tunnel. Most people see dyslexia as a disabling condition that is likely to have far reaching, negative effects on the lives of those existing with the condition; this book attempts to change that attitude and encourages understanding that starts with what the individual is *good* at. The book explores what many with dyslexia do well, and in some instances is unique to the way that the dyslexic brain works. Eide and Eide encourage us to open our minds to another view of dyslexia, and put a great analogy forward of looking through a telescope the wrong way, then we only see a narrow and pinpointed vision of the world, hold the telescope the other way and then we get a connected, broad framed, global picture of the view.

This is a well-written text by two eminent neuroscientists, who put forward well-researched ideas backed by valuable evidence from selected research papers from across the world. The text concludes with practical advice for those who are dyslexic and those working with individuals with dyslexia, to capitalise on the advantages that come with this condition.

References

Cancer, A, Manzoli, S and Antonietti, A (2016) The alleged link between creativity and dyslexia: identifying the specific process in which dyslexic students excel. *Cogent Psychology* 3(1).
Companies House (2019) *Virgin Enterprises Ltd.* www.beta.companieshouse.gov.uk/company/01073929 (accessed 02. 12. 19).
Department for Education/Department of Health (2015) *Special Educational Needs and Disability Code of Practice 0 to 25: Statutory Guidance for Organisations which Work with and Support Children and Young People who Have Special Educational Needs or Disabilities.* https://assets.publishing.service.gov.uk/government/uploads/system/uploads/attachment_data/file/398815/SEND_Code_of_Practice_January_2015.pdf (accessed 20. 12. 19).
Davis, RD (1997) *The Gift of Dyslexia.* London: Souvenir Press.
Eide, BL and Eide, FF (2011) *The Dyslexia Advantage: Unlocking the Hidden Potential of the Dyslexic Brain.* London: Hay House UK Ltd.
Forbes (2019) *Billionaires: The Richest People in the World.* www.forbes.com/billionaires/#68a8910f251c (accessed 02. 12. 19).
Hayes, C (2018) *Developmental Dyslexia from Birth to Eight: A Practitioner's Guide.* London: Routledge.
Intelligence and Security Committee of Parliament (2018) *Diversity and Inclusion in the UK Intelligence Service.* London: House of Commons, OGL.
Jung-Beeman, M (2005) Bilateral brain processes for comprehending natural language. *TRENDS in Cognitive Science* 9: 512–518.
Logan, J (2010) *Unusual Talent: A Study of Successful Leadership and Delegation in Dyslexic Entrepreneurs.* London: City University London, Cass Business School.
Made by Dyslexia (2018) *The Value of Dyslexia: Strengths and the Changing World of Work.* London: Ernest and Young.
Mourgues, CV, Preiss, DD and Grigorenko, EL (2014) Reading skills, creativity and insight: exploring the connections. *The Spanish Journal of Psychology* 17.
Nicolson, R (2015) *Positive Dyslexia.* Sheffield: Rodin Books.
Rooke, M (2016) *Creative Successful Dyslexic: 23 High Achievers Share Their Stories.* London: Jessica Kingsley.
Schneps, M (2015) *Dyslexia can Deliver Benefits.* www.scientificamerican.com/article/dyslexia-can-deliver-benefits (accessed 19. 07. 19).
Scott, R (2004) *Dyslexia and Counselling.* London: Whurr Publications.
Sun, Y, Lee J and Kirby, R (2010) Brain imaging findings in dyslexia. *Paediatrics Neonatal* 51(2) 89–96.
Treffert, DA (2014) Savant Syndrome: realities, myths and misconceptions. *Journal of Autism and Developmental Disorders* 44: 564–571.
Williams, EL and Casanova, M (2010) Autism and dyslexia: a spectrum of cognitive styles as defined by minicolumnar morphometry. *Medical Hypotheses* 74: 59–62.
Wolf, M (2008) *Proust and the Squid: The Story and Science of the Reading Brain.* Cambridge: Icon Books.
World Economic Forum (2016) *The Future of Jobs: Employment, Skills and Workforce Strategy for the Fourth Industrial Revolution.* www3.weforum.org (accessed 20. 12. 19).

9 Research and academia

> Everybody is a genius. But if you judge a fish by its ability to climb a tree, it will live its whole life believing that it is stupid.
> (Usually attributed to Einstein but the origin is debatable)

Introduction

Scientific research into dyslexia has burgeoned dramatically in the last fifty years. This chapter will consider the cost of research that has been undertaken thus far, and the difficulties of raising money for such research. It will examine the value of research into the workings of the brain and neuroscience, and how this has potentially benefited a range of difficulties that go far beyond the remit of information processing differences (IPD): genetics, hearing, immunology, etc.

In this chapter you will be introduced to the use of technology, such as functional magnetic resonance imaging (fMRI), positron emission tomography (PET) and electroencephalograms (EEG), making research into dyslexia far more reliable than the largely qualitative research conducted in the past. Through questions and reflective material, you will be encouraged to debate the cost of such technological research, and how its use has increased, compared to only twenty years ago, when most of the research was conducted as qualitative, comparative style studies. This type of research requires the use of more neuroscience-based researchers, with access to expensive, specialist equipment and advanced skills and knowledge to interpret the findings; you will be asked to consider where that leaves the single postgraduate researcher.

The workings of the brain

One of the greatest challenges in the twenty-first century is to research the workings of the brain, which has long been an intriguing mystery to humans. The brain is a unique organ in the human body and the one most admired and most questioned over the centuries, and probably the most enigmatic: it has been described as science's ultimate frontier. Over the years scientists and medical personnel have investigated and dissected other organs of the body, often using animal experimentation to interpret what they see; in this way they have been able to understand the mechanics of the heart, lungs, liver, kidneys, etc. It is even possible to successfully transplant these organs from one individual to another and, with ever increasingly sophisticated technology, prosthetic limbs can allow people to walk, and to live with artificial hearts, kidneys, livers, etc. The brain, however, has remained the outstanding mystery and no machine or other human intervention has been found to replace the brain or even do a fraction of what it does at the speed at which it does it. Despite massive advances in knowledge and understanding of the brain and how it works, any form of brain surgery remains extremely dangerous, and requires infinitesimal accuracy and enormous skill to perform. This has been compounded by the fact that anything to do with the brain has historically been caught up in a tangled culture of mystique, magic, religion and ethics.

A brief history of our understanding of the brain and its workings can be seen in Figure 9.1 but of course, there were many other worthy contributors to this story and too many to include them all here.

Considering the complexity and continuum of dyslexia, and the manner in which it pervades so many areas of human development, in so many ways, it is vital that we move our conception of IPDs away from one-dimensional explanations, into a multi-dimensional explanation of cause. The difficulty for the researcher is that it eventually means close co-operation between many research factors, as no one person or research project can possibly have the knowledge, understanding and facility to look at all these areas together. This means that they have to know about research going on across the world and in other research facilities, and then have access to these facilities, and be able to make connections between the differing projects and their findings, like a giant, complex jigsaw. Without this level of co-operation, work in this area is unlikely to progress at any pace, as each research facility works alone and in ignorance of what could be important discoveries being made elsewhere. This is immensely wasteful of financial resources and of the enormous talent of those working in this field.

In 2003 there was a huge leap in scientific knowledge with the sequencing of the human genome. This is potentially the gateway to understanding so much more about human development, evolution and the future direction of medicine; it could potentially open the way to an understanding of the whole wiring system of the brain and neurophysiology. Some geneticists believe that one day gene therapy could eliminate genetic disease and neurodevelopmental conditions, and in the case of dyslexia could indicate the children at risk of IPDs, and thereby enable appropriate intervention strategies to be put in place from birth, to both understand the condition better and to support its many challenges. However, the immense scale of the datasets obtained will take many years into the future to interpret and understand, this has been acknowledged and supported by Europe's Human Brain Project. This ten-year project, started in 2013, aims to build a research infrastructure to advance all aspects of brain research. There are six research platforms within the Human Brain Project (HBP, 2013).

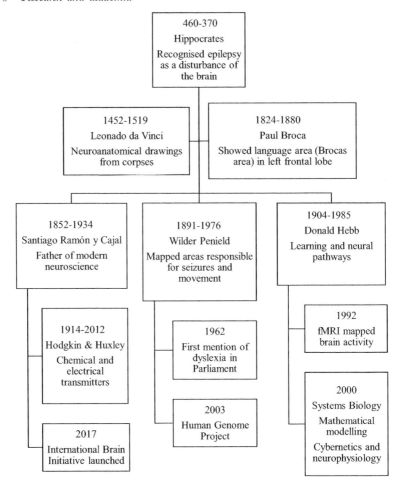

Figure 9.1 Brief history of the understanding of the brain

1   *Neuroinformatics.* This is the field of research which deals with the organisation of neuroscience data. The idea is to bring together data from numerous research institutions in a professionally managed web-based forum, with the intention of acquiring new information, to enable it to be shared, stored, published, analysed, modelled, visualised and simulated. This would be a platform for the open and honest sharing of neuroscience data through a knowledge exchange network, to ensure that important research projects have the best and most up-to-date information for their further research into treatments and interventions for brain related diseases and conditions. This would particularly be helpful to the smaller, and often isolated, but incredibly important, research projects with often a lone researcher.

2   *Brain simulation.* This involves the replication of brain structure and anatomy through computer models. This could also involve Deep Brain Stimulation (DBS), where a device, similar to a pacemaker, is inserted into the brain to deliver electrical impulses to specifically identified areas that are thought to be responsible for particular functions. This could also involve placing electrodes on to the outside of the scalp, to stimulate and produce chemical and functional changes within the brain.
3   *High-performance analytics and computing.* This is the use of high-performance computing to analyse large data sets looking for patterns, comparisons and differences. Each human brain probably has hundreds of billions of neurons, connected by thousands of trillions of synapses and this allows you to get some idea of the scale of the immense task for any researcher. Many complex research projects are potentially threatened by the ability to manage the high volumes of data that they generate, potentially denying valuable and important research funding being awarded, and strands of research potential from emerging. Developing tools to investigate neuronal circuits is vital to the future success of this type of research.
4   *Medical information.* This area of the HBP (2013) attempts to negotiate access to confidential patient data and identification of conditions and diseases. Neuroscientific research is a highly sensitive area of research with many ethical, moral, cultural and religious hurdles to overcome. Before research can begin that involves humans or animals, it is imperative that ethical approval is obtained for the credibility of that research. This means placing before a panel of peers and seniors the details of the conduct and reasoning behind that research and any potential benefits. This is required to protect the participants from accusations of harm to their safety, dignity and rights, but also to protect researchers, who might be accused of manipulation of the participants. An ethics committee is usually made up of lay people and professionals, independent of the research and of any financial sponsors of that research, and their role is to consider the potential benefits of that research, evaluate the methodology and check for informed consent. Each ethics committee is likely to place different criteria for access to material such as patient medical records, and to have particular issues of patient confidentiality and privacy. This variation makes compliance difficult and very long winded. Such difficulties can lead to a negative impact upon the quality of research, as compromises have to be made. The UK Policy Framework for Health and Social Care Research (NHS, 2018) sets out principles of good practice to protect patients, whilst at the same time attempting to enable patients and service users to participate in research. This framework also has to ensure that researchers understand how to remain within the context of the law, without needless bureaucracy. However, there is a plethora of organisations and regulatory bodies potentially involved, such as the General Medical Council, General Dental Council, General Pharmaceutical Council, Health and Care Professions Council, Human Fertilization and Embryology Authority, Human

Tissue Authority, and many more. All these interested parties make any research in this area a very difficult ethical path to tread.
5   *Neuromorphic computing or neuromorphic engineering.* This is the development of brain inspired computing. This research intends to replicate the nervous system of the human body, the production and use of neural networks, taking the form of the brain and artificial intelligence.
6   *Neurorobotics.* The use of robots to test brain stimulation, this combines neuroscience with robotics and artificial intelligence, by replicating with computers the biological neural networks and brain inspired algorithms.

From the details of this one project the complexity of this research area can be seen, and it requires the ability and willingness of all these disciplines to come together to interpret the complex information that each of their research areas bring about. This bringing together and sharing of research findings could potentially bring about new knowledge and a better understanding of how science can inform practice in the future. Many of these disciplines heavily overlap, so communication between them is vital to learning more about the complexities of the working of the brain. It is essential that in the future information from biology, chemistry, genetics, biochemistry, medicine, psychiatry, psychology, engineering, mathematics, computing and many other disciplines talk together and they, in turn, share that information with educationalists, teachers, practitioners and clinicians, to better inform their practice with those who are affected by these conditions.

Research can be ground breaking, revolutionary and trailblazing, but it can also lead to blind alleys and become obstructive. That is not to say that well-founded and well-constructed research, even when it apparently leads nowhere, is wrong; often it is discovering what is *not* is as useful as discovering what *is*. However, Featherstone (2017) reminds us that the internet probably reaches up to four billion users, and that, together with the pace of neuroscience which has escalated beyond all comprehension in the last twenty years, means that any reader or interested party needs to treat all research with *professional caution,* as many of these research projects are badly written up, inadequately researched and biased, which can generate what she calls 'neuromyths'. It is certainly the role of a researcher to read everything with caution, and to question everything, including material that has been conducted by eminent researchers and regarded as 'gospel' over many, many years. This is certainly not to say that you throw the baby out with the bath water, and not all older, previously accepted research is wrong and not all new research is correct: simply a healthy regard for question and analysis is required for a reliable researcher, in the light of advancing knowledge.

Researchers are often out to make a name for themselves, and with the current pressure on university staff to research, publish and increase the profile of their university, the financial status of their university and often their jobs are on the line. This could potentially afford a conflict of interest between sound, reliable research (which takes time, often considerable expense and expertise), causing misinterpretation and misapplication, and a concern with making a 'quick buck'. Obtaining adequate funding for longitudinal studies, which may take many years to come to fruition, is always difficult, and the finance departments of universities and research institutions want headline grabbing results to increase their profile and attract more students to their establishments. They want results and they want them *now*!

Having set in place these warnings and understanding the importance of questioning everything that we *thought* we knew, many older established ideas, theories and principles are still valuable and need to be built upon (Featherstone, 2017). In the same way that not all older established theory is wrong, so many new ideas can become 'fads', and are in danger of being picked up by institutions as a quick fix, and a way for them to generate more income for themselves. An example of this might be the notion of 'learning styles' and the concept that we all learn in a particular way. Certainly, there are many different ways to learn, but these are usually context specific, and learning to change a wheel on the car may require different ways to learn than learning to appreciate art or drama, but the idea that we all have a preferred learning style is questionable (Hayes, 2018). This whole concept has generated numerous commercial companies expecting to make money from educational institutions to assess their students/pupils, each company with a differing term for each, so-called, learning style ranging from two to over seventy.

> if we view each learning style as dichotomous (e.g. visual vs. verbal) that means that there are 2 to the power of 71 combinations of learning styles … more than the number of people that live on the earth.
> (Jarrett, 2015, p. 208)

Some colleges and universities have tested all their new intake for their preferred learning style, at immense cost to the establishment and probably very little return to either the student or the educational establishment. Some large companies, particularly in America, make huge profits selling testing programmes and training consultants to colleges across the world, with no really robust research to back up their claims.

Another area of suspect research is that of colorimeter testing and coloured overlays, supplying coloured lenses to children with dyslexia, when the benefits of this are probably very limited. Evans and Allen (2016) conducted a systematic review of the research into this area and found that whilst they may alleviate some of the symptoms of visual stress it is certainly not likely to be of any great benefit to those with dyslexia.

Other contenders for the title 'neuromyth' would be programmes such as the Dore programme and Brain Gym. These programmes claimed to offer a 'quick fix' for those with learning difficulties, at a huge cost to vulnerable parents, desperate to do everything within their power to help their children, taken in by grandiose claims that have no research-based verification. Many parents paid over £1,500 for their child to be enrolled on the Dore programme and over

£500 each for inclusion on the Brain Gym system, which are considerable sums, and out of the financial reach of many families. Many of the improvements identified could simply be the result of a placebo effect which has not been fully investigated.

Conkbayir (2017) suggests that one reason for these expensive neuromyths is the present lack of coordination of research between disciplines, and a lack of collaboration between professionals. She suggests setting up a public online forum for research proposals but recognises the difficulty of knowing the reliability and validity of the research posted to such a forum, and the challenge of disseminating that complex material to the general public in a format that they would find accessible. Another suggestion from Conkbayir (2017) is for increased accessibility to online articles, journals, research databases and libraries, free of charge. This could currently mean a significant loss of income to the original publishers, and ultimately to the researchers and writers. However, it is possible that this could be compensated for by the research community, universities and research institutions acceptance of advertising. This is a highly controversial idea which needs to be discussed in the academic world (possible solutions and fire walls would need to be put in place), but currently subscriptions and pay walls are a major barrier to the single researcher, providing little access to article directories and repositories.

Qualitative versus quantitative

Research generally falls into three classifications: qualitative research, quantitative research (sometimes called the positivist and interpretivist research traditions) and a mixed methods paradigm, which broadly is a merging of the other two. However, research rarely falls exclusively into either qualitative or quantitative. And until recently most educational research and research into dyslexia and IPDs has been of a qualitative nature. Often the perception of qualitive research is that it is too subjective and lacks an element of objectivity; qualitative research is often seen as exploratory, acting as a precursor to more rigorous quantitative research. The advantage of qualitative research is the ability to study topics which are descriptive and hard to quantify, like social and emotional issues, feelings and states of mind. Qualitative research can be conducted in a naturalistic setting through observation, with an opportunity to explore holistic experience.

In general terms qualitative research can be classed as interpretivist, involving words and observations, based in social reality, as distinct from quantitative research, involving numbers, measurements and a whole way of thinking of gathering data in a numerical format. A mixed methods paradigm, however, combines the strengths of qualitative and quantitative, potentially compensating for the weaknesses of both methods.

REFLECT ON THIS

1 Classify the following research topics into either qualitative, quantitative or mixed methods paradigms (Table 9.1).

Table 9.1 Types of research

	Quantitative	Qualitative	Mixed methods
a			
b			
c			
d			
e			

    a   How do children in year seven, who have been identified with dyslexia, feel about their 'label'?
    b   How many children in a particular local authority currently have an Education, Health and Care plan?
    c   Children who are poor readers, engaged with Reading Recovery, achieve significant benefits at the end of the twenty-week programme?
    d   A case study of two children identified with dyslexia, to gain an in-depth understanding of their learning needs.
    e   Seven-year-old children with reading delay will role play more aggressively than children without.

2   How difficult did you find it to be so definitive with your classifications and why?

Research in practice

There does appear to be a large chasm between researchers in the field of neuroscience and the practitioners working closely with children each day, whether in nurseries, schools, play centres, the homes of childminders or parents. Talking to practitioners indicates that many believe that neuroscience is too complex and complicated to be of any relevance to them in their practice; they do not understand it and the difficult technical and medical terminology, and they are unable to make the links between early brain development and the holistic development of the child that they see before them. Scientists and researchers may have little or no practical experience of working with 'real' children, or their experience is historical, and their association with academia makes it hard to disseminate their knowledge in an accessible format (Figure 9.2).

The more that practitioners who work with young children know and understand about brain development, and the neuroscience behind that development, the better they will be able to understand and support the children in their care and the impact upon learning. Practitioners need to feel confident to use neuroscience to inform their practice, but this will probably

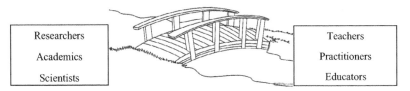

Figure 9.2 Bridging the chasm from researchers to practitioners

require a considerable financial investment in training, and committed, knowledgeable professionals to drive this through. One recommendation of the Royal Society (2011) report was that all initial training and continuing professional development for teachers and practitioners should have a module about neuroscience or at least an element of it within them, which can be directly related to practice.

> Educators face formidable obstacles learning from relevant research, including a lack of background knowledge and technical vocabulary; inability to access scientific journals; and school demands that often focus attention on day-to-day coping. The average educator, even one with an interest in neuroscience, rarely hurdles the obstacles to access, analyse, and digest relevant brain research. Typically, educators (and parents) are at the mercy of attention-grabbing headlines and entrepreneurial ventures and products exploiting a flourishing brain-based, evidence-based market niche.
>
> (Pugh and McCardle, 2016, p. 45)

Strong links need to be made between the research community and those at the 'coal-face' but particularly for those working with those in special needs, at all ages. Such links can be beneficial to both the practitioners and the researchers as those working day by day with individuals with IPDs can inform, critically evaluate and discuss the effects of new technologies and possibly direct further research in a particular direction, enabling knowledge to flow in both directions. However, before this could happen all interested sides need to build a common vocabulary of understanding, and this is likely to pose a significant challenge.

Cost vs benefits ratio

Any research proposal needs to consider the cost vs benefits ratio, that is, a consideration of likely benefits achieved, for the work and financial investment made. Benefits could be the discovery of crucial findings, which could potentially lead to significant advances in a particular field. It can be difficult or even impossible to predict whether or not significant findings will be discovered, and, as has happened in the past in science, the most influential findings can occur by chance. Examples of this would be Leo Baekeland in 1907 who discovered the world's first plastic (Bakelite), whilst researching in another field entirely. The microwave oven was invented by Percy Spencer in 1945, when investigating radar equipment and X rays were also a product of accident by Wilhelm Röentgen in 1895, even the pacemaker by Wilson Greatebatch in the 1950s. In a search for the elixir of life, Chinese alchemists discovered gun powder, and the most famous accident of all was Alexander Fleming in 1928, with the discovery of penicillin, after a holiday allowed mould to contaminate his cultures. All these examples could probably be attributed to luck!

The researcher, when putting forward a research proposal, needs to weigh up whether there are cost benefits to society, whereby failure to undertake the research could disadvantage human potential. As can be seen this type of balancing of the books can be extremely difficult to predict, as even the best and most well-planned research can finally yield no new or significant knowledge. However, it must also be considered that in the long term a negative result can be as important as a positive, managing to rule out the myths, the false positives and the false negatives.

> Current brain research offers a promissory note, however, for the future. Developmental models and our understanding of learning will be aided by studies that reveal the effects of experience on brain systems working in concert. This work is likely to enhance our understanding of the mechanisms underlying learning.
>
> (Santiago Declaration, 2007)

> Education affects the wellbeing of individuals and has economic benefits. The economic and social cost of an education system that does not facilitate learning for all and learning throughout life is high.
>
> (Royal Society, 2011, p. 1)

Brain imaging

As important as the technology for brain imaging is, it is still not possible to identify the presence of dyslexia in an individual from the images produced, although some researchers in America, led by Professor John Gabrielli from the Massachusetts Institute of Technology, believe that they could be close to achieving this. However, the technology is rapidly increasing the researchers' and scientists' knowledge of how the brain works. It is quickly becoming a reality to map the areas of the brain and identify the locations most important for complex tasks such as reading, and to detect any abnormalities and differences within both the structure and importantly the functionality of the brain.

The safe use of magnetic resonance imaging in the 1990s was a huge advance and allows researchers to see changes in the developing brain.

154 Research and academia

- Magnetic resonance imaging (MRI) uses radio waves, magnetics and computers to produce an image of the body and its soft tissues, unlike X rays which image bone and hard tissue with the use of radiation and can be critically dangerous to other cells and tissue.
- Functional magnetic resonance imaging (fMRI) is also radiation free and measures changes in blood oxygenation and flow that can occur in response to neural activity.
- Functional near infrared spectroscopy (fNIRS) is a non-invasive measure of blood flow (haemodynamic) within the brain, thereby measuring brain activity and differences.
- Positron emission tomography (PET) scans can be used to produce 3D images of the brain to work out how well the brain is functioning and identifying anomalies with the use of radio tracers which detect the amount of radiation emitted. The higher the activity of a specific brain area, the larger the quantity of glucose (or oxygen) consumed and the more radioactive substance is accumulated.
- Computerised tomography (CT scans or CAT scans) use X rays and a computer to generate images which are usually only used if an anomaly has already been detected.
- Magnetic resonance spectroscopy (MRS), also known as nuclear magnetic resonance spectroscopy (NMRS), measures biochemical and metabolic changes within the brain.
- Magnetoencephalography test (MEG) records brain activity at the time of functioning. This is used extensively as a research tool in neuroscience to check the brain's response to specific external stimuli and to map specific areas of the brain for reading, communication and language development and other functions.
- Diffusion tensor imaging (DTI) maps the directional movement of water molecules in the brain, searching for microstructural differences along neural tracts.
- Electroencephalogram (EEG) is a recording of brain activity and tracks the electrical activity in the brain, and how brain cells are communicating with each other through electrical impulses.

Clearly this 'run down' of some of the available brain imaging technologies is very rudimentary, and my apologies to those who know so much more about this than I do, but gives some indication of the complex research tools available to neuroscientists studying IPDs in the brain. Each of these technologies will require experts to administer, analyse and evaluate their evidence, but is likely that these (and those that will come after them) will eventually be able to unlock the mystery of how we use our brain to read, communicate and learn language. Such advanced imaging equipment can be used for so much more and is used regularly in medicine to preserve and save lives, but use in experimental research into the brain will be invaluable to future understanding of this mysterious organ that we call the brain.

The cost of such equipment is immense with a probable NHS investment in scanning equipment set at over £460 million and individual machines costing between £579–£1.4 million each so the use of such equipment for research purposes becomes enormous; add to this the expertise to analyse and evaluate the images and the scale of the use of such equipment becomes clear. Individual scans can cost between £84 and £1,000 each.

The cost of research has to factor in a number of items:

- Equipment and materials either bought or hired
- Travel to other research establishments, interviews and investigations, etc.
- Use of space in research areas
- Time costs of researchers and assistants
- IT and infrastructure
- Lighting, heating, etc.

REFLECT ON THIS

With a colleague, discuss some of the following questions.

1. Does the ability to use technology and quantitative methods of research now negate the need for qualitative methods of research in this field?
2. How do you think that neuromyths become accepted as truths? How dangerous do you think this is to the future of research in this area?
3. What limitations are there to brain imaging procedures?
4. How can the use of such images be helpful to practice with children with IPDs?

Chapter reflections

The exact nature of how the brain works in those with an IPD is still to be discovered, but further research into neuroscience will almost certainly eventually bring about a more accurate identification and mapping system. Dyslexia is certainly a lifelong condition, but many people seem to be able to compensate for it and become high functioning dyslexics, able to read and work in employment which requires organisation and structure. Greater understanding derived from valid and reliable research may well ensure that more of these with dyslexia can function adequately within a reading society.

Structural and functioning neuro-imaging has helped already to advance knowledge, but the problem with dyslexia is that there is never going to be one single gene or one single cause found to account for it; there is no single gene that makes one a reader or not, and it is more likely that there are multiple causes all leading to the same thing, what Hans Driesch (1867–1941), the German biologist, called equifinality. This is the concept that the same end state can be reached from many different directions, with biology and the environment impacting the brain in an epigenetic interrelationship. The biggest challenge has to be whether through the medium of neuroscience and neuroimaging, children from a very young age can be identified *before* reading and literacy become a problem. It could be that in the future effective intervention could involve manipulation of functional brain plasticity artificially (that is how the brain changes in response to learning), or even genetic engineering, to increase adaptability and prevent dyslexia from occurring in children and babies that are at risk. Of course, some will say that this is the stuff of science fiction and there are many, many ethical and moral barriers to such thinking, even if it were desirable which is dubious.

> There are inspiring developments in basic science although practical applications are still some way off.
>
> (Royal Society, 2011, p. v)

The Royal Society reminds us that greater understanding of the working of the brain obtained through inspiring neuroscience could help many individuals to become more contented, more healthy and more productive members of society, enabling them to contribute significantly to the financial and social elements of humanity.

> A neuroscience perspective recognises that each person constitutes an intricate system, operating at neural, cognitive and social levels, with multiple interactions taking place between processes and levels.
>
> (Royal Society, 2011, p. 17)

Further reading

Featherstone, S (2017) *Making Sense of Neuroscience in the Early Years*. London: Bloomsbury Publishing.

For those who know very little about neuroscience and feel intimidated by the very complexity of the word, this is a great introductory guide. This book deals with the myths and legends of what the brain can and can't do and of the various truths that we have accepted over the years which are now looking less and less likely, with the explosion of new research findings.

In easy-to-read terms this book helps to unravel some of the complexities of this area of knowledge. The book focusses on babies and young children and stresses the importance of those working with the very youngest children knowing how advances in neuroscience must shape their practice.

References

Conkbayir, M (2017) *Early Childhood and Neuroscience: Theory, Research and Implications for Practice*. London: Bloomsbury Academic.

Evans, JW and Allen, PM (2016) A systematic review of controlled trials on visual stress using intuitive overlays or the intuitive colorimeter. *Journal of Optometry* 9(4): 215–218. www.ncbi.nlm.nih.gov/pmc/articles/PMC5030324/ (accessed 21. 08. 19).

Featherstone, S (2017) *Making Sense of Neuroscience in the Early Years*. London: Bloomsbury Publishing.

Hayes, C (2018) *Developmental Dyslexia from Birth to Eight: A Practitioner's Guide*. Abingdon: Routledge.

Human Brain Project (HBP) (2013) www.humanbrainproject.eu/en/about/overview (accessed 20. 08. 19).

Jarrett, C (2015) *Great Myths of the Brain*. Chichester: Wiley-Blackwell.

NHS (2018) *UK Policy Framework for Health and Social Care Research*. www.hra.nhs.uk/planning-and-improving-research/policies-standards-legislation/uk-policy-framework-health-social-care-research/ (accessed 20. 08. 19).

Pugh, K and McCardle, P (2016) *How Children Learn to Read*. Abingdon: Routledge.

Royal Society (2011) *Brain Waves Module 2: Neuroscience Implications for Education and Lifelong Learning*. London: The Royal Society.

Santiago Declaration (2007) http://www.santiagodeclaration.org/ (accessed 25. 08. 19).

10 The great dyslexia industry

Introduction

Just a quick look at any *Dyslexia Contact* magazine (the official magazine of the British Dyslexia Association), and you will find it filled with adverts for equipment, paraphernalia, therapies and courses, designed to make the life of the person with dyslexia easier or even to overcome dyslexia entirely. Dyslexia has become big business, a money-spinner for quick fixes, therapists, schools and education. Unfortunately, it is possible that, for some vulnerable people, they may be being preyed upon by charlatans with their money-making scams. In the last twenty years an entirely new industry has emerged, the *dyslexia industry*, which some say relies on the uncertainties of the definition and identification of the condition. However, for many these inventive and creative aids and support are invaluable to enable them to compete on equal terms with their non-dyslexic colleagues, school friends and workmates.

Parents, teachers and practitioners are often confronted by the mass of equipment and resources that are available to those with considerable cash to spend; just one look online will reveal that, for a price, there are hundreds of aids out there from coloured paper to dictionaries, from digital voice recorders to exam reader pens. It could be that dyslexia has become a condition that only the rich can afford.

This chapter will briefly investigate some of the claims of the manufactures and will illustrate by talking to those who have invested their hard-earned cash into these products their effectiveness.

My own son was identified as being dyslexic over twenty-five years ago. He attended a mainstream primary school and was becoming more and more disruptive and difficult to manage in the classroom. He really struggled to read, and I was told that he was just lazy and probably not very bright, as, despite their best efforts, he still could not read effectively. When I suggested that perhaps he was dyslexic I was disregarded and told that there was no such thing as dyslexia, only fussy parents and lazy children! This felt as though they were abdicating all responsibility for the teaching of my son, placing 'the blame' for his difficulties squarely upon the shoulders of the child and the parents. At great cost I took him each week to a reading tutor, who believed that she could help, but she too told me that there was 'no such thing as dyslexia'. When eminent people such as Professor Julian Elliot, a Chartered Psychologist from the University of Durham and Fellow of the British Psychological Society, were also saying that there is no such thing as dyslexia, people tended to take note and in an interview for the Daily Mail newspaper, in 2014, Elliott described dyslexia as:

> A meaningless label used by middle-class parents who fear their children are being branded stupid.
>
> (Elliott: reported by Macrae 2014)

Even the politicians joined in the debate, with Graham Stringer (Member of Parliament for Blackley, Manchester) calling for the 'dyslexia industry' to be killed off, describing dyslexia as:

> A cruel fiction ... No more real than the 19th century scientific construction of 'the æther' to explain how light travels through a vacuum, he argued that the reason why so many children struggled with literacy was because they had been failed by the educational 'establishment'. Rather than admitting that poor instruction was at fault, he argued, a brain disorder called dyslexia had been invented.
>
> (Elliott and Grigorenko, 2014, p. 1)

Dyslexia at this time was sometimes dubbed 'the middle-class disease', suggesting that working-class children did not have the condition. No parents want their child labelled 'thick', stupid or lazy, especially as this appears to call into question the standard of their own parenting skills. The suggestion was that this was articulate, professional parents making excuses for their children's difficulties, and precisely because they were so articulate, and knew how to 'work' the system, they could obtain additional support for their children that the less articulate and well-educated parent was unable to achieve. From this can be seen that the very concept of dyslexia and information processing differences (IPDs) was brought into question with parents, professionals and experts alike unable to agree. This is not to suggest that there is any attempt to deliberately mislead but as a quotation from the late, great John F. Kennedy depicts often it is an acceptance of what has become an apparent fact after years of peddling a particular logic.

> The great enemy of the truth is very often not the lie, deliberate, contrived and dishonest, but the myth, persistent, persuasive and unrealistic.
>
> (Kennedy, 1963, p. 471)

Science versus subjection

The report by the Royal Society (2011) suggests that neuroscience is crucial to any advancement of educational practice in the future, to understanding how humans learn and consequently to an understanding of how to teach. This idea brings with it both advantages and disadvantages, and an opportunity to examine in fine detail *how* we teach. This brings the authenticity of science to education, which until recently was seen as a social and behavioural area of study, built largely upon theory and subjective judgement. The very word 'science' brings with it a suggestion of objectivity and numerical research, rather than observational opinion, bringing with it the perception of a greater sense of credibility and reliability, which is likely to be largely welcomed by the educational community. However, with this clamour for credibility has come a wealth of commercial interest from those hoping to create financial wealth from the promotion of their goods and services. Unfortunately, sometimes this is founded upon the concerns of loving families wanting to do the 'best' for their children, and often they are struggling to understand why their child is not learning in the way that they expect with the traditional teaching methods. Teachers and educationalists have also fuelled this commercial explosion, realising that their tried and tested pedagogy is not always appropriate for all children, and keen to increase their knowledge and improve their teaching. Headteachers, local authorities and politicians can also be sucked into areas of an inappropriate and unproven commercial industry, with the drive to improve grades, SATS results and Ofsted ratings, in an effort to increase their potential funding and investment.

Undoubtably the stakes are high: a 'quick fix' or sudden improvement of results can even change party political politics, after all, we would probably all vote for a party that could ensure that all children could read successfully and reach their full potential in life.

> There is already a glut of books, games, training courses and nutritional supplements, all claiming to improve learning and to be backed by science.
> (Royal Society, 2011, p. 18)

However, as the Royal Society report suggests, such an enormous volume of information coming from such a vast range of sources makes it extremely difficult to see the 'wood from the tress', and to see what is 'real' science and what is pseudo-science. This needs to be based on reliable and valid evidence, independently assessed and accurately ascribed to well-founded, defensible sources, not based on commercial interests and pecuniary intention.

Whether they are bona fide rigorous researchers or hoaxers and charlatans, there is a hugely profitable industry out there for the 'quick fix', the one fairy-tale pill, miracle therapy or magic wand that *cures* this condition. However, as you have read in previous chapters of this book, this is highly unlikely and any treatment, intervention or product that seems too good to be true probably is. It is likely that these genetically based conditions (which we are born with and stay with us to the grave) can never be completely cured, and by using the term 'cured' it is medicalising the condition, and putting it in the same category as a disease, which given the right medication can usually be healed, so that the individual will no longer need to be identified with that label. Whilst those with an IPD can be helped and supported to manage their life around their learning differences, it is highly unlikely that they could ever be said to be cured.

Appropriately supporting those with an IPD needs to be done with skilful and insightful teaching and empathetic support from family, friends and mentors. The problem with this approach is that it is slow, painstaking and often monotonous; it is not headline grabbing and 'zinggy'. However inspiring and creative a teacher may be when they try to impart skills and knowledge, it is likely to involve a great deal of repetition, for consolidation, in a variety of differing formats, through rehearsal to automaticity. The skilled and enthusiastic teacher will take close account of the learner's feelings and experiences, able to generate enthusiasm and engage them with their learning by building upon existing knowledge and understanding. It is likely that each one of us has encountered a teacher such as this at some point in our lives, if we are lucky there will have been more than one, but it is also just as likely that we have encountered teachers who have poor people skills, poor communication and have just not understood what is required of a highly motivated, committed professional. As a teacher of many years standing, I frequently heard the comment from teachers that *I have been teaching all day and s/he has still not learned anything*, but the very definition of the verb *to teach* is embedded in learning: you cannot be teaching if someone is not learning. There is no such thing as the perfect teacher, but the teacher that strives to understand their charges and their learning needs is committed to improving their own teaching techniques and can inspire, motivate and build on what the learner already knows, to develop their feelings of self-worth and confidence to take on further learning.

Whilst it is important to remain open to new ideas, new therapies or pedagogies, it is vital to remain cautious, viewing all such *miracles* as controversial and suspect, especially if they come with a high financial price tag. As with all research it is vital to consider the reliability and validity of any intervention, to assess its credibility, and that it is carefully scrutinised before being implemented or deployed. Some tests of credibility may be helpful:

- *Stability* – The intervention needs to stand the test of time, and any progress seen today should at least be seen to be stable or enhanced by tomorrow, in a month and even in two years' time, often called external consistency.
- *Reliability* – The intervention needs to produce the same results each time that it is administered. This can be internal or external reliability. To be an internally reliable intervention it needs to produce the same results in two equally matched samples delivered at the same time (split half). To be externally reliable the measure is between one use and another, in a test/retest method.

- *Validity* – The results need to measure what the research claims that they measure.
- *Content validity* – The results claimed for the intervention may not represent the whole programme/intervention, they may only relate to parts of it, and thereby skew the results of the whole.
- *Sensitivity* – The programme/intervention may not work as well with all people, and there may be significant variables in the sample that can influence the results. All people are different and a programme/intervention could possibly be influenced by the make-up of the sample, their age, gender, location, ethnicity, culture, socio-economics and many other variables some of which may be highly localised.
- *Conceptual framing* – The programme/intervention needs to be set within the context of previous research in the field, both positive and negative. It is important to understand where this sits within the conceptual jigsaw.
- *Transparency* – The openness and honesty of the proponents of the programme/intervention must be apparent in the findings. Any research into the product must have raised questions about its credibility and integrity and these need to be reviewed and validated.
- *Funding* – The source of funding for the research into the product must be transparent. For example, if a product, such as a particular chocolate bar, is to be investigated for the number of people who put it as their favourite confectionary, but the research for this is funded, whole or in part, by the manufacturers of that same product, there is a serious conflict of interest and potential for bias, as the makers have a financially vested interest in having research results that look positively on their product.
- *Cogency* – The conclusions of any research into the programme/intervention need to be firmly rooted in, and supported by, the results.
- *Sample* – The evidence for any success of the programme/intervention may be based on a single research study, but these results need to have been confirmed by widespread studies with large sample sizes. The selection of the sample/s needs to be clearly indicated and rigorously designated. Whilst it is not possible to stipulate what is a *large enough* sample (this will vary according to the population), there is no doubt that the findings will be considerably strengthened by repetition and corroboration. A small uncorroborated study is unlikely to be seen as a strong body of evidence.

These are ten indicators to look for when assessing the credibility of research; they do not comprise an exhaustive list but do offer suggestions for areas to be aware of when attempting to ascertain the credibility of claims made for particular products. Table 10.1 offers suggestions for evaluating the strength of that evidence:

Table 10.1 Evaluating the overall strength of the evidence

Levels of credibility	What to look for	What does this mean?
Very strong credibility	High quality evidence. Tested on large samples. The samples are inclusive of differing ages, cultures, socio-economic groups, locations, ethnicity and gender, etc. Reliable and valid with consistent and stable findings. Peer reviewed research exists. Any research has been independently conducted and does not rely on funding from the proponents.	You can be confident that this programme/intervention/equipment does or does not have the effect claimed by the proponent.
Strong credibility	Some high quality evidence. Tested on a large enough sample. The sample is inclusive of differing ages, cultures, socio-economic groups, locations, ethnicity and gender, etc. Reliable and valid with mostly consistent and stable findings. Peer reviewed. The research has been independently conducted and does not rely on funding from the proponents.	You can be reasonably confident that this programme/intervention/equipment does or does not have the effect claimed by the proponent. It is important to continue to be aware of new evidence coming to the forefront.
Moderate credibility	Moderate quality evidence. Generally consistent results. Some evidence from the samples may not be as diverse as it could be. Apparently reliable and valid with a level of consistency to show generally stable findings. The research may be funded or part-funded by a proponent of the programme/intervention/equipment.	The programme/intervention/equipment may or may not have the effect claimed by the proponent. There are reasons to suspect that the evidence offered could be skewed or biased. Continue to be aware of new evidence coming to the forefront.

(*Continued*)

Table 10.1 (Cont.)

Levels of credibility	What to look for	What does this mean?
Limited credibility	Moderate to low quality evidence. Small or limited sized samples possibly lacking diversity of context. Inconsistent results with research unable to be replicated. Reliability and validity may be compromised. The research is likely to have been funded or part-funded by a proponent of the programme/intervention/equipment being examined.	The programme/intervention/equipment may or may not have the effect claimed by the proponent. The evidence displays some significant shortcomings. It is likely that contextual difference may substantially affect the outcomes. It is vital to continue to be aware of new evidence coming to the forefront.
No credibility	No credible evidence exists.	There is no plausible evidence that the programme/ intervention/equipment has any effect either positively or negatively.

Adapted from Department for Internal Development (2014)

The powers of suggestion

Many of the 'get fixed quick' interventions are probably built upon a number of well-founded psychological phenomena, many of which are well known to the rigorous researcher, and it is vital that steps are taken to eliminate or account for them in the research.

- *The placebo effect.* This is about the immense power of suggestion when, unbeknown to a person with a particular condition or disease, a 'sugar pill' or other chemically inactive treatment (a small sweet or Smartie), is administered and triggers apparent recoveries. This is thought to arise when the individual truly believes that a particular intervention is going to work, and this imitates real physical and neurological changes. There is no doubt that to the patient this recovery appears to be real, and this further enhances their belief in the placebo. Over the years this phenomenon has been observed and researched extensively.
- *Hawthorne effect.* This controversial effect refers to the idea that when under observation, people behave differently. We all behave differently when we know that we are being watched, few of us pick our nose or scratch ourselves in public, but it is perfectly normal behaviour, that we all do. This effect can be short term but it can also result in statistically significant effects, which may be positive or negative, and skew results of research. This may result from the novelty of having a researcher observing and working with a subject, or could be due to a demand characteristic, that is, subtle cues from the investigator of the results they are expecting to see. This is an attentional effect with individuals reacting favourably to an intervention, just because they feel that they are the centre of attention.
- *Pygmalion effect.* When teachers or parents expect a child to show significant improvement, these children do exactly that – a self-fulfilling prophecy is in action. In this motivational effect, individuals feel special, and this may make them try harder and thereby improve quite naturally regardless of the intervention.
- *Halo effect.* This is a bias whereby a researcher's judgement can be influenced, either positively or negatively, by other characteristics, for example, if the subject is bubbly and articulate a teacher may judge them to be more able than they actually are. Alternatively, the child who is shy and retiring and does not communicate well can sometimes be assumed to have more difficulties than they actually do.
- *Baffled by science effect.* This is seen when a researcher is 'blinded' by science, that is they are more prepared to accept something as true, when it is accompanied by technical vocabulary from neuroscience. Experiments conducted by Weisberg et al. (2008) showed that people were more ready to believe an explanation which contains words related to neuroscience, even when they are irrelevant to the explanation. The scientific language can even mask the really salient information. Commercial companies can

be very alluring with their language, to persuade the consumer to purchase, and by applying a thin veneer of research credibility to their products, can draw in the unsuspecting parent or school.
- *Matthew effect.* This is the progressive widening of the gap between those who are good at a particular skill and those who are not so good, due to the differences in experience and exposure to that skill, in other words accumulated advantage. This may be because a child who finds reading difficult is likely to read less, thereby reducing their exposure to print still further; this is likely to increase the gap between them and their peers. This is exacerbated when they need to read in order to learn and it creates difficulties in all other subjects so that they fall further and further behind.

Such prevailing powers of suggestion can significantly skew research in surprising ways. This is evident in the millions of pounds spent each week by multi-national companies on advertising. However much we may like to think that we are immune to the power of advertising – *it won't affect what I buy* – these adverts are designed to feed into our subconscious with associations and interpretations. Many of us will buy a more expensive advertised brand, rather than a cheaper supermarket own brand, believing it to be superior, even though the contents may be the same. TV advertising is manipulating our behaviour through the power of suggestion.

REFLECT ON THIS

> The results of this study do not suggest the abandonment of using educational technology, but rather that impartial experimental research and judicious assessment of its effectiveness in education are essential to balance the efforts invested in promoting and embellishing these innovations ... Because economic interests and sensationalized media naturally drive the publication and dissemination of studies showing positive, significant differences ... a balance in publication is necessary.
>
> (McDaniel and Fraser, 2014, p. 12)

1. Consider the quotation from McDaniel and Fraser (2014) above. How far do you agree with their assessment?
2. How easy or otherwise do you think it is for a practitioner to obtain and evaluate the evidence presented for a particular intervention?
3. How much do you think that the economics of research impact firstly what is researched and secondly the results?

Nutritional and dietary supplements

There are many claims for the success of nutritional and dietary supplement interventions for a range of IPDs, including dyslexia. Eating a wholesome balanced diet is essential to human mental and physical development, but perhaps something as simple as 'popping a pill' a day could help to alleviate some of the difficulties experienced by those with dyslexia. Numerous studies exist which have examined the effects of nutritional deficiencies in and intolerances of salicylates, food additives, food colourings, flavourings, refined sugar, zinc, iron, magnesium, vitamin B12 and vitamin D. Other chemical allergies and intolerances have also been researched briefly. However, the one most associated with neurodevelopment and dyslexia is the addition of fish oil to the diet, that is, Omega-3, Omega-6 and Evening Primrose oil (eicosapentaenoic acid (EPA), docosahexaenoic acid (DHA) and Gamma Linolenic Acid (GLA)). These are highly unsaturated fatty acids and claims by some of the manufacturers have been made that significant changes in metabolism have been observed when added to the diet of those with dyslexia. However, the evidence for any improvement in reading is, according to Zelcor and Goldman (2015), very inconsistent and limited. They call for more controlled, randomised studies to be conducted and, in particular, to consider what might be an optimum dosage, over what period of time and at what stage of development.

One set of trials in 2007, conducted by the local authority in Durham in collaboration with Oxford University, involved administering Omega-3 fish oil capsules to 3,000 school children from a range of socio-economic backgrounds, to help to raise their GCSE grades. Unfortunately, the results were rather inconclusive, and the experiment has since been castigated by many researchers including Goldacre (2008) as poorly designed research.

There is no doubt that Omega-3 is certainly big business: go to any large supermarket and you will find a large array of fish oil supplements on sale in their aisles. The market research firm MarketResearch.com (2019) estimated, in a report in 2019, that Omega-3 products were worth £116 million in Britain alone, and worldwide probably as much as £426.877 million!

Computer assisted programs

There have been many reviews of computer assisted technologies and their usefulness for those with IPDs, but most have revealed inconsistent findings (Archer et al., 2014; Cheung and Slavin, 2012; etc). One such popular program is Word Shark, which has a drill-and-practice approach to learning and is designed to improve reading and spelling levels; it is well used by many schools in the UK. Interestingly there appears to be only one positive published evaluation of this program by Singleton and Simmons (2002), from the psychology department at Hull University. In this study the main finding was that the children enjoyed using the programme, and 96% reported feeling more motivated to learn to read and spell because of the novel imagery and mnemonics. However, Crook and Lewthwaite (2010) showed that this initial enthusiasm could be short lived, and any significant long-term improvement was not, in their study, supported by the empirical evidence, even with programmes that have real-time communication (RTC). Their research appeared to raise a number of questions about the mixture of results, particularly about the 'dosage' or duration of the intervention and its significance. Singleton and

Simmons (2002) did find that teachers reported findings that there was significant improvement in their pupils' reading and spelling. However, a PhD thesis by Longstreet (2014) brought these findings into question, believing that Singleton and Simmons (2002) relied too heavily on teacher opinion, and their research design was fundamentally flawed, as they also needed to obtain data from children who actually used the programme.

> The subjective opinions of teaching staff derived from questionnaire measures and were not supported by objective, empirical findings.
> (Longstreet, 2014, p. 6)

She concluded that computer assisted technology generally produces only small and moderate effects on reading and literacy. This conclusion was also reached by McDaniel and Fraser (2014) in a more comprehensive study of computer assisted technology, delivered in a paper to the American Research Association. Messer and Nash (2018) concede that computer assisted learning, if effective, would be a very cost-effective method of teaching children with reading delays, but agree with McDaniel and Fraser (2014) that it is often not as valuable as the program creators claim. According to Messer and Nash (2018), there are very few randomised controlled trial evaluations for these programs, and the ones that there are find that there are some small gains in reading, but these are often minimal.

> Thus the weight of available evidence suggests that most computer-based interventions are not of substantial help to children with reading difficulties.
> (Messer and Nash, 2018, p. 142)

This same evaluation also suggests that it could be that the subject matter of *reading* does not lend itself to this form of teaching, as opposed to subject areas with more factual content. There is also a very real controversy about whether it is easier to read in a digital format (on a computer screen or handheld device), or in an 'old fashioned' book-based format. Whilst there is much to be said for both, Horvath (2019) suggests that, for learning, a printed book is probably more effective. In digital format the reader can change the font, increase the size of the print and even change the colour of the text and the background, which may be especially useful to those with dyslexia; however in a digital format the print is continuous, and does not have a fixed spatial location, which can improve memory. Horvarth (2019) found that when reading short passages there was no difference between reading from a screen and reading from a book, but when reading longer passages, print almost always outperforms digital. He explains this by referring to the brain's spatial representation system, which allows you to recognise when something in a room has been moved or removed, even when you are not sure what.

Print ensures that material is in an unchanging and everlasting three-dimensional location. This is why even though we rarely focus on the spatial organisation of paragraphs, many can recall that a particular passage is 'about halfway through a book on the bottom righthand page'. This unvarying location is embedded within our memory and can be utilised to trigger recall of relevant content in the future.

(Horvath, 2019, p. 37)

No computer program, however good, can really provide the personal and instantaneous feedback that is vital to the successful learner. However, computer assisted programs can possibly be beneficial to children at risk of reading difficulties, if combined with good access to real-time books, and the children can obtain the social and emotional support to boost levels of motivation and task perseverance. Whilst such programs, and other computer assisted learning devices, cannot replace interaction with the traditional teacher, they may supplement such teaching, and become an additional learning tool alongside a close home and school collaboration. No computer program or electronic device claims to 'cure' dyslexia and most concentrate on the aspects of dyslexia related to reading, numeracy and literacy rather than attempting to look at dyslexia more holistically as an IPD.

Movement-based therapies

Movement-based therapies, such as Brain Gym, the Dore programme (which went into liquidation in 2008), Dyslexia, Dyspraxia Attention Treatment (DDAT), Retained Reflex Syndrome, Primary Movement and the Mulhall Integration Programme, are many and various, but all are essentially based on the idea that physical exercise can reconnect and redirect electrical circuits in the brain, and develop an immature central nervous system. Unfortunately, there appears to be little hard scientific evidence that they produce the results that their commercial proponents claim.

Brain Gym was developed by Paul Dennison in the 1970s. It consisted of twenty-six activities requiring motor control, balance, laterality and co-ordination. This is a programme which has been purchased by many schools up and down the country. Brain Gym teaches teachers to direct the exercise programme, at a cost of between £275 to £600 per teacher, and before practising they must pay to be a member of Edu-K, the authorised membership body of Brain Gym in the UK. Brain Gym International is found in over eighty different countries across the world and is registered as a non-profit organisation. However, Brain Gym is also big business, as it makes money through training licences and selling branded books and resources. Schools and colleges can also pay their consultants to work with their children, students and staff.

In 2007, Hyatt reviewed five studies evaluating Brain Gym, and concluded that there was no scientific evidence to support the programme. Goldacre (2008) suggests that those who have bought into Brain Gym have been blinded by the apparently bogus neuroscience explanations for the way it works. However it is possible to see that there are some very basic premises for Brain Gym which are really sensible, such as increasing levels of systematic exercise, taking regular breaks, ensuring appropriate body hydration and a well-balanced healthy diet ... but surely these are obvious!

The Dore programme was based on the idea that children with dyslexia have cerebellar developmental delay, and by invigorating one area of the brain it will improve other areas, but there is no available evidence that suggests that any improvement in one domain (motor skill development) can lead to improvements in other domains (reading and cognitive development). Parents paid over £2,000 for the programme, which lasted two years and required those embarking on the programme to travel to the centre in Manchester regularly, thereby incurring the cost of travel and time from work. There certainly appears to be no reliable research evidence to back its claims of a 'miracle cure' for dyslexia. There was one heavily criticised report by Reynolds et al. (2003), which concluded that the programme was associated with significant and lasting improvements in reading. Rack et al. (2007) later gave a powerful critique of the research methodology for the Reynolds et al. (2003) investigation, and concluded that the results were heavily flawed.

Case study

Robbie is now twenty-six years old, but at the age of eight was assessed for dyslexia. He hated school and now describes what went on there as bullying, not only by his peers but also the teachers. He concedes that this was probably due to ignorance of the condition, but cannot forget the feelings that this brought to him. His family were desperate to help him and to try all that they could to ensure that he could learn to read and write. Robbie describes his writing as 'chicken scrawl' and said that his one aim was to be able to read his own writing, he says that he would write down his notes for school, but when he came to read them back they meant nothing to him. He also described difficulties with his balance and visual discrimination. Robbie described how he always compared himself to his sister, who did not have the problems that he did.

Robbie's mother was a nurse and a lecturer, and she heard about the Dore programme and how it had helped other children in the same situation. With the help of other members of the family they managed to scrape together the £2,000 investment required to start the programme, and embarked on over two years of travelling from North Wales to Manchester every two months, which was a considerable financial outgoing. This meant Robbie having time away from school and someone in the family taking time from work to accompany him. Robbie received tremendous support from his grandparents and, with the family support, undertook the exercises that the programme required religiously, even taking some of the equipment (there was a lot of this) with them on holiday so that they could maintain continuity. Each session lasted approximately two hours.

The programme was a combination of talking therapy and exercise, with large balls to balance and catch, wobbleboard balance, work sheets, reading practice, etc. It was explained to Robbie, by the programme's co-ordinators, that the exercises were to help to direct the neural pathways and thereby to improve automaticity.

Robbie now works in engineering and still describes feelings of panic when asked to read. A major problem that he has to cope with, on a day-to-day basis, is his level of organisational skill, but he has developed his own strategies for dealing with these. He still lives at home, and still receives support from family and friends. He believes that there are still significant prejudices in the workplace, and that at times he still comes across bullying in the form of hurtful comments and behaviours; however, he has learned to deal with these and overcome them. He now understands that his difficulties are far more complex than simply literacy related, and that his condition spans the whole spectrum of IPDs.

Robbie believes that the Dore programme helped him significantly, and was delighted when he achieved his ultimate aim of being able to write intelligibly enough for him to be able to read his own writing. He expressed his gratitude to his family for investing in him financially, through time and by supporting hm to undertake the exercises as instructed.

Another movement-based programme is Primary Movement which is based on the idea of retained primary reflexes. This is the concept that we are born with reflexes which are crucial to the survival of the newborn (sucking, rooting, startle, Moro, etc.), but these would normally 'switch-off' as the child develops, and they no longer become essential to survival. This theory suggests that for some children this 'switch-off' does not occur, making it difficult to develop to norm as they are impeded for example by the clenching of the muscles of the hand and neck for writing etc. This programme demands that participants undertake the prescribed exercises for ten minutes every day for 9–12 months. Trainers for this programme undertake eight days of training with the company at a cost of approximately £1,250.

REFLECT ON THIS

There is no way of knowing whether the improvements that Robbie and his mother described in the case study above were directly related to the exercises from the Dore programme, or simply relate to maturational and developmental change. Clearly, he had immense support from a loving family, and you have already read in this text about the importance of stable mentorship to the self-esteem of those with an IPD.

1   Could the Hawthorn effect and the power of suggestion have influenced the apparent improvements that Robbie describes?
2   Programmes and interventions such as the Dore programme are very expensive and this does mean that only those with such funds available to them, are able to access this type of support. Work with a colleague to consider the implications for this on equality, diversity and inclusion.

Perceptual disturbances

It must be apparent to all that if a person cannot see properly then they will find reading, writing and spelling extremely difficult, so any person who is suffering from any kind of eye strain or visual disturbance needs to visit a qualified optician and, if appropriate, to wear suitably adjusted spectacles, contact lenses or overlays. However, claims have been made that those with dyslexia could be suffering from visual disturbances. This is not to say that they cannot see the print, but that the print appears distorted in some way, due to sensitivity to certain wavelengths of light, what is referred to as Scotopic Sensitivity Syndrome. The type of distortions experienced could be that words appear to move around on the page, letters reverse, the background to the print can be seen as too bright and even pulsating; this is often known as visual stress. These distortions can lead to very slow and inefficient reading, headaches, extreme fatigue when reading and, understandably, a general unwillingness to read.

Irlen (1991) put forward the idea that by using coloured overlays and lenses this perceptual difficulty can be eliminated. She stressed that this is not a replacement for good teaching of reading but will enable the sufferer to access the reading material more effectively. Helen Irlen persuaded an optical manufacturing laboratory to produce a device known as an Intuitive Colorimeter which had a variety of different coloured filters in different tones and intensities. This enables a suitably qualified optician to assess the colour and intensity which a particular individual would find most helped them to read and would prevent the visual distortions that they experience when reading. This whole concept that colour can improve reading has spread rapidly throughout education possibly because this is apparently such a simple and cheap way to improve reading and to demonstrate a commitment to diversity and inclusion. I don't suppose that there is a school, college or university in the country that does not advise its teachers and lecturers to put some students' notes on coloured paper, despite the fact that Irlen (1991) admits that there is an almost unlimited number of possible colours and hues and it is likely that only a colour specific to an individual is going to produce the improvements claimed. If this is to work the colours need to be carefully and diagnostically prescribed by a vision specialist, with appropriate training. Irlen (1991) herself admits that she does not know why the coloured filters work.

> it is possible that the filters selectively reduce specific, troublesome wavelengths of light.
>
> (Irlen, 1991, p. 57)

Visual stress related to dyslexia is highly controversial but Singleton and Henderson (2007) found that 41% of children in their sample, with dyslexia, were also identified with visual stress, compared to 23% of a non-dyslexic control group. This study also appeared to show that the children with dyslexia gained significantly higher reading rates when using coloured overlays. However, although there appears to be initial evidence that overlays help reading, more recent studies such as Henderson et al. (2013) and Ritchie et al. (2012) have suggested that they do not, and that there are serious methodological issues related to the initial research.

> Possibly one of the reasons for this lack of explanation is that the very nature of visual stress syndrome and of its role in reading has been questioned and therefore the entire enterprise might just be a false trail.
> (Uccula et al., 2014)

Interview

The following interview shows Lawrence's experience of coloured filters and coloured lenses. Lawrence is now in his early thirties and having been in the army is now successfully employed in 'civvie street'.

> When I was eleven, I was taken to the opticians to go on the colourimeter machine. She put on lots of different filters on the machine and asked me to read a piece of writing. When a certain colour came up the writing did seem clearer. However, I am not sure whether the glasses that they made for me with the colour made any difference to my reading at all. It sort of dulled the page, but it also made everything the same colour, somehow it was not as bright, a bit like sunglasses. The coloured filters that the teachers gave me were not really of any advantage.
>
> I don't think that anyone picked on me for wearing them or bullied me, but the teachers were always shouting at me to wear them. The trouble was that I was always losing them. My organisational skills were just not good enough to remember to have them with me whenever I needed to read. It was not like wearing glasses when you are short sighted, so when you get up in the morning you need to put your glasses on to see things, so there was no natural reminder. It's just not 'cool' to wear glasses and when I went to college at sixteen, I did not wear them. In the end I just lost them completely!

There is clearly quite an industry based around the concept of visual stress, selling overlays, lenses and coloured glasses, often also associated with consultations costing families many hundreds of pounds as these glasses are not available on the NHS.

Optometric vision training, sometimes called vision therapy, is about training the eye muscles to focus and direct the eyes to coordinate and function efficiently, but is more than just muscle control and aims to look holistically at the child, involving working with balance and co-ordination by using wobbleboards, eye tracking equipment, balls and hula hoops. Clearly if a person has difficulty focusing the eyes on the print before them, this is going to be tiring, and they will find it difficult to concentrate, a fundamental prerequisite for successful reading. To enable reading a child must be able to move their eyes smoothly along a line, back and forth, and to jump from the end of one line to the beginning of another over an extended period of time; if this is difficult their motivation to read will be low. This becomes self-fulfilling as the less they practice reading the harder they will find it.

This is a highly controversial therapy, not supported by the Royal College of Ophthalmologists, and in 2009 a review by Barrett, found no significant evidence that visual therapy could substantiate the claims that it makes for those with dyslexia and other IPDs (Barrett, 2009).

Chapter reflections

The investigations into these 'get fixed quick' interventions have suggested that many have not been reliably evaluated in scientific studies, and there is limited research, not only into their effectiveness but also more worryingly into their safety, health consequences and dosage. In some cases, they are being administered by untrained, unqualified, inexperienced and uninsured practitioners.

> In theory, anyone can set themselves up as a 'therapist' and charge fees with very little, if any, experience. You only have to log on to the internet or read a newspaper to find lots of so called 'universities' advertising degrees in almost anything in exchange for a fee. The problem is that these certificates can look very real!
>
> (Chivers, 2006, p. 17)

Any decision to engage with a particular intervention needs to be based not on testimonials and internet advertising websites, but on objective information and solid research evidence. At the moment it should be of great concern that money is potentially being taken from concerned parents and cash-strapped schools and put into the coffers of private companies, when the research base for their products may be untested and limited. Whilst all these interventions are likely to place considerable financial strain upon families, schools, local authorities and governments, huge emotional strain can be placed on the children and their families, as they conceivably experience repeated failure and possibly delay more effective interventions from being put in place. If a family has invested several thousands of pounds into a programme, whether intentional or not, there will be an expectation upon the child that they may not be able to accede to, and this can create tension and anxiety which in turn could impede learning and further increase a feeling of low self-esteem.

There are a huge number of commercial enterprises competing for a very limited pot of money in education: they are appealing to a growing interest in research-informed practice, and see this as one way to make their products stand out; however, without rigorous and informed scrutiny of this research we can be fooled into acceptance. In a culture of high stakes accountability schools will inevitable want to invest in something they are told will increase their grades and

Ofsted ratings. However, money spent on ineffective interventions is money that is no longer available for interventions that really can make a difference; such interventions may not have the 'razzmatazz' of some of the commercial products, but the weight of good solid research evidence still indicates that intensive and creative reading teaching, with an emphasis on phonics training, undertaken by specialist, trained and qualified teachers, is the most appropriate way forward.

Further reading

Chivers, M (2006) *Dyslexia and Alternative Therapies*. London: Jessica Kingsley Publishers.

Whilst this is not a new book, it is quite unlike any other text about dyslexia. Chivers writes in an easy style and tackles issues relating to alternative therapies in a down-to-earth and sensible manner. Whilst I cannot say that I would agree with all that Chivers writes, it is certainly a text which provides food for thought, whether you agree with it or not. She attempts to provide a balanced account and to remain objective throughout her investigation of over fifty alternative therapies, but she entreats the reader to keep an 'open mind'. Chivers admits that many alternative therapies have not received the rigorous scrutiny that perhaps they should have, but that anecdotal evidence from those who have engaged with them is strong.

References

Archer, K, Savage, R, Sanghera-Sidhu, S, Wood, E, Gottardo, A and Chen, V (2014). Examining the effectiveness of technology use in classrooms: a tertiary meta analysis. *Computers & Education* 78: 140–149.
Barrett, B (2009) A critical evaluation of the evidence supporting the practice of behavioural vision therapy. *Ophthalmic and Physiological Optics* 2: 4–25. www.ncbi.nlm.nih.gov/pubmed/19154276 (accessed 29. 12. 19).
Cheung, AC and Slavin, RE (2012). How features of educational technology applications affect student reading outcomes: a meta-analysis. *Educational Research Review* 7 (3): 198–215.
Chivers, M (2006) *Dyslexia and Alternative Therapies*. London: Jessica Kingsley Publications.
Crook, CK and Lewthwaite, S (2010). Technologies for formal and informal learning. In Littleton, K, Wood, C and Staarman, JK (eds), *International Handbook of Psychology in Education*. Bingley: Emerald.
Department for International Development (2014) *Assessing the Strength of Evidence*. www.assets.publishing.service.gov.uk/government/uploads/stystem/uploads/attachment_data/file/291982/HTN-strength-evidence-march2014.pdf (accessed 11. 12. 19).
Elliott, J and Grigorenko E (2014) *The Dyslexia Debate*. New York: Cambridge University Press.
Goldacre, B (2008) *Bad Science*. London: Fourth Estate.
Henderson LM, Tsogka N and Snowling MJ (2013) Questioning the benefits that coloured overlays can have for reading in students with and without dyslexia. *Jorsen* 13: 57–65.

Horvarth JC (2019) Are print books better for learning than digital texts? *Times Educational Supplement*, 6 September.

Hyatt, KJ (2007) Brain Gym building stronger brains or wishful thinking. *Remedial and Special Education* 28(2): 117–124.

Irlen, H (1991) *Reading by the Colours: Overcoming Dyslexia and Other Reading Disabilities.* New York: Avery Publishing Group.

Kennedy, JF (1963). *Public Papers of the Presidents of the United States: John F. Kennedy, 1962*, Whitefish, Montana: Literary Licensing. LLC.

Longstreet, K (2014) *Wordshark: A Computer-Assisted Programme.* PhD Thesis: University of Southampton. www.blog.soton.ac.uk/edpsych/files2015/09/Wordshark-Dec-2014-Katie-Longstreet.pdf (accessed 20. 12. 19).

Macrae F. (2014) Dyslexia is a 'meaningless label used by middle-class parents who fear their children are being branded stupid', professor claims. *Daily Mail*, 26 February.

MarketResearch.com (2019) *Global Omega-3 Concentrates Market by Manufacturers, Regions, Types and Application Forecast to 2024.* www.marketresearch.com (accessed 20. 12. 09).

McDaniel DC and Fraser, BJ (2014) *Effectiveness of Integrating Technology across the Curriculum: Classroom Learning Environments among Middle-school Students.* Paper presented at the annual meeting of the American Educational Research Association (AERA), Philadelphia, PA,April 2014. https://www.academia.edu/9335598/Effectiveness_of_Integrating_Technology_across_the_Curriculum_Classroom_Learning_Environments_among_Middle-school_Students (accessed 12. 12. 19).

Messer, D and Nash, G (2018) An evaluation of the effectiveness of computer-assisted reading intervention. *Journal of Research in Reading* 41(1): 140–158.

Rack, JP, Snowling, MJ, Hulme, C and Gibbs, S (2007) No evidence that an exercised based treatment programme (DDAT) has specific benefits for children with reading difficulties. *Dyslexia: An International Journal of Research and Practice* 13(2) 97–104.

Reynolds D, Nicolson R and Hambly H (2003) Evaluation of an exercised based treatment for children with reading difficulties. *Dyslexia: An International Journal of Research and Practice* 9: 97–104.

Ritchie, SJ, Della Sala, S and McIntosh, RD (2012) Irlen colored filters in the classroom: a 1-year follow-up. *Mind. Brain Education* 6: 74–80.

Royal Society (2011) *Brain Waves Module 2: Neuroscience: Implications for Education and Lifelong Learning.* www.royalsociety.org (accessed 20. 12. 19).

Singleton C and Henderson L (2007) Computerized screening for visual stress in children with dyslexia. Dyslexia: An International Journal of Research and Practice 13 (2) 130–147.

Singleton C and Simmons F (2002) An evaluation of WordShark in the classroom. *British Journal of Educational Technology and British Educational Research Association* 32(3): 317–330.

Uccula, A, Enna, M and Mulatti, C (2014) Colors, colored overlays and reading skills. *Frontiers in Psychology* 5: 833. www.ncbi.nim.nih.gov/pric/articles/PMC4114255/ (accessed 29. 09. 19).

Weisberg, DS, Keil, FC, Goodstein, J, Rawson, E and Gray, JR (2008) the seductive allure of neuroscience explanations. *Journal of Cognitive Neuroscience* 20(3): 470–477.

Zelcor, M and Goldman RD (2015) Omega-3 and dyslexia: uncertain connection. *Canadian Family Physician (CFP)* 61(9): 768–770. www.ncbi,nlm.nih.gov/pmc/articles/pmc4569108/ (accessed 20. 09. 19).

11 Politics, politics and policy

Introduction

The final chapter, and conclusion of this book, will examine the social and political context for dyslexia within a culture. It will explore the whole concept of the politicisation of dyslexia with both a small and a large P and consider whether the funding provision required to support those with dyslexia is currently sufficiently adequate and how this can only be changed with the support of both national and local governments. This chapter will look at the return on investment of appropriately supporting our children with dyslexia in terms of reduced unemployment benefits being paid, significant reduction in the numbers within the criminal justice system or those requiring support from social services and the NHS. This is frequently brought about by, as Boden (BDA, 2019b) suggests, *throwing away dyslexia talent*. This waste of potential could almost be seen as criminal, wasting money and often destroying lives.

> We're throwing away dyslexia talent and there's no good reason why. It's costing us money, hurting businesses and leaving young people with fewer opportunities.
>
> (Boden; BDA, 2019b, p. 4)

Historical context

A brief review of the history of information processing differences (IPDs), and in particular dyslexia, shows how there has been a constant struggle for these conditions to be recognised in official circles from the days of William Pringle Morgan, in the early part of the twentieth century, and his concept of word blindness, to the present day when dyslexia is officially recognised as a disability within the *Special Educational Needs and Disability Code of Practice: 0–25* (DfE/DoH, 2015). The hunger of employers for ever more literate and better educated employees has increased exponentially over recent years, and a new report (DfE, 2019) showed that in 2017–2018, 50.2% of all young people experienced higher education, which was the declared vision of Prime Minister Tony Blair (1997–2007) in his famous 'Education, Education, Education' speech. The importance of literacy to successful life outcomes has become more and more apparent and society clearly needs more productive workers if the UK is to be able to compete within a global context.

The first real breakthrough in the recognition of dyslexia as a particular learning difference was made in 1987, when the prime minister of the day (Margaret Thatcher) spoke about the need for dyslexia to be recognised and made important enough for educators to be aware of. By 1997, and the advent of a Labour government after eighteen years of Tory prominence, the funding for special educational needs, including dyslexia, was extended and research interest increased as more generous research grants were made available. However, since that time an economic recession has occurred, and financial austerity in all public-sector areas has been prevalent, resulting in some back sliding, even causing some local authorities, such as Warwickshire County Council, to announce that they do not recognise dyslexia as a discreet condition and any different from general low literacy (Henshaw, 2018). Warwickshire education authority stated that children would no longer be assessed for dyslexia, as the teaching techniques for general poor readers was the same as those with dyslexia. This is tantamount to saying that although the techniques have not worked to this point, we will give them more and more of the same and then they WILL learn! Fortunately, the policy makers of Warwickshire have since been forced to withdraw this very poorly thought through guidance.

In the past the willingness to recognise dyslexia and other IPDs has been brought about by a lack of firmly agreed definition, and any way to definitively identify the conditions in an individual. This lack of agreed definition is still largely applicable today and is possibly the cause of some of the unwillingness, on the part of governments, to provide the required resources to tackle the issues and support the children. Even as late as 1972, the Tizard Report indicated their scepticism about the existence of developmental dyslexia as a discreet condition (Tizard, 1972) and in 1978 Baroness Warnock (DES, 1978) mentioned the pressure placed upon her by senior civil servants to omit dyslexia from her report, presumably due to the fear of the resulting financial implications. Even today the debate goes on about the 'myth' of dyslexia with Elliott and Nicolson (2016) ferociously debating this contentious area.

It was not until the 1980s that dyslexia was firmly recognised by the government as a Specific Learning Difficulty (SpLD), and funding was made more available, with statements of educational need being made for those appropriately assessed and identified.

Politicisation

The whole business of literacy and reading is always high on the agenda of any government and any suggestion that there might be a 'quick fix' for reading for the 16.4% of adults in England alone who can be described as having 'very poor literacy skills' is likely to make an easy headline for the press and news media. To put this into context this is approximately 7.1 million people or one in six people in the population; in Scotland that rises to one in four; in Wales one in eight and one in five in Northern Ireland (National Literacy Trust, 2017). Such headline material can be the difference between an electable political party and a non-electable one, as reading really is at the centre of what we currently see as success in education, and education is at the centre of most of our achievements as a society. For this reason, it is an area which has become highly politicised, both in terms of party politics and the politics of everyday decision making or the micro-politics of life.

Socio-economic divisions are entrenched in UK society and according to the Office for National Statistics (2019) some indications of poverty, such as poor housing, childcare and food, are increasing year by year, and this has become of national concern. Politicians use education, and in particular literacy, as the key to both societal success and financial success, which brings with it the potential to improve society for all, to even out the 'haves' and the 'have nots' and to promote a more inclusive and equitable society … this is election gold dust! However, whilst politicians of all parties agree that education is the route to equality and social justice, what they cannot agree upon is how to achieve it. Despite this there is a symbiotic relationship between politics and education, whereby politics affects education and education affects politics.

Accountability

Governments demand value for money, rightly so, as they are entrusted with our hard-earned cash to provide an equitable society for us all to live in. To this aim governments require measurable results, as do schools and parents, and there is nothing wrong with this. The problem arises when it comes to measuring these results, and even the debate over what we mean by 'results'. What may appear to be a good result for a parent and individual child (which might be measured in levels of self-esteem, resilience and happiness) may be very different from a 'good' result for a particular school, or even between schools (which might be measured in terms of reading scores and Ofsted ratings).

> The measure of progress can depend upon how one views the purpose of education and the means of achieving that purpose.
> (Reid, 2016, p. 260)

Reid (2016) talks about the possible conflict of purpose and means of education, and how this conflict can impact the need for accountability. For politicians, accountability means testing, benchmarks and league tables, enabling numerical measurements to divide schools and local authorities into high and low performing areas. It must be accepted that the public purse is not unlimited, and some form of fiscal constraint is always going to be inevitable.

> the reality of market forces and accountability of the public purse may determine the nature of the educational process in schools and the educational experience of children in the classroom.
>
> (Reid, 2016, p. 260)

The public purse is of course a limited resource and there are so many worthy causes impacting upon it. This puts each cause into competition with each other, as if one gets more it is inevitable that the others get less. However, imagine a situation where there was the introduction of research-based IPD screening tests, in the early years, with robust predictive rates, which could lead to proactive support and intervention for children at risk, thereby closing any processing gaps before a sense of failure sets in. This could potentially prevent many children from suffering reading frustration, educational disadvantage and catastrophic collapses of self-esteem and self-worth. This in turn could continue into adolescence and adulthood, with potential reductions in antisocial behaviour, criminal activity, reductions in mental health issues and suicides, reduction in social care support and relief to the benefit system and subsequent savings to the public purse and drain on the economy. This becomes a win-win situation allowing more funding to be available to the many other worthy causes that are currently desperate for more public funding. Such a policy, which would need to be initiated by government and rolled out across the country, could be a resource-effective and cost-effective means of using public funding to the benefit of all in society. An initial outlay, could, if explained in these terms, be a popular political and party-political voting attraction, and could bring huge savings to the economy.

Inclusion policy

Humans by their very nature appear to need to group things together and to classify themselves according to common factors: these may be age, religion, ethnic origins, gender, etc. Any difference from that group can present a difficulty for the members of the group. In 2013 Nutbrown et al. suggested that a policy of inclusion is often based upon location, whether the children are sharing the same space; certainly this was the premise of the Warnock Report (DES, 1978), which saw the closing of hundreds of special schools in England in favour of as many children as possible being educated within main stream schools. However, as Nutbrown et al. (2013) suggest, this is not always appropriate, and a policy based entirely upon location is doomed to failure, as it is not necessarily meeting the needs of the child. Nutbrown et al (2013) showed that a policy of inclusion is more about an attitude of mind, and working to eliminate prejudice, injustice and inequality. This implies a radical reflection upon our own selves and our own lives.

> The task, then, is to enact inclusive policies in practice that challenge our preconceptions about human beings; children and their families; society and success and failure themselves.
>
> (Nutbrown et al. 2013, p. 3)

Some might argue that literacy is at the heart of the life chances of individuals, and this is probably true, but it cannot be seen as cause and effect. An individual's life chances are related to so many other interrelated aspects, including genetics, parental interest, physical environment and location, health, diet, socio-economics and social exclusion, etc. It is unlikely that simply by putting in place policies to improve inclusion and the teaching of literacy society will be able to overcome these difficulties and ensure equality of opportunity. Reid (2016) reminds us that so much more needs to be accomplished:

> While inclusion can be seen as a desirable outcome in terms of equity, it can also be seen as a threat and creates a potential conflict between meeting the needs of individuals and establishing a framework that has to meet the needs of all.
>
> (Reid, 2016, p. 260)

REFLECT ON THIS

> Inclusion is about a radical deal more than physical location.
>
> (Clough, 1998, p. 5)

1 Consider whether any of the children in your setting are physically included in terms of location, but, because of an IPD, are excluded from particular elements of the setting. For example, do some of the children with reading difficulties have to miss certain sessions or play periods in order to have their reading support?
2 How could this be addressed by inclusive thinking?

Collaboration

IPDs are multi-faceted and therefore require a holistic and multi-professional approach to support. This is recognised in the Common Assessment Framework (CAF) (DfCSF, 2009) in England, which acknowledges that support for children with special educational needs probably needs to come from more than one agency, and transition arrangements need to be in place between these agencies as a child matures and moves through the system. Bringing together professionals from a range of different disciplines will inevitably be challenging within an inclusive environment. The concept of a team around a child is not new, and probably goes back to the start of formal education in the early nineteenth century when schools were as much about offering a place of safety and better health care as well as learning. In more modern times, Prime Minister Tony Blair launched the paper *Every Child Matters* (DoH, 2003), which really brought forward the concept that some form of collaboration or partnership between agencies and services might improve outcomes for children and their families.

In order to achieve the best outcomes for children with IPDs, it is vital that all professionals who work with these individuals and their families communicate well together, engaging with a partnership approach. Not only is there the potential for this to save money on resources, and workload, but time can be used more effectively with less duplication, and the messages conveyed can be more consistent and reliable, thereby reducing the numbers of potential misunderstandings. However, a conflicting view came in a review of multiagency working by Atkinson et al. (2007), which suggests that some professionals working in multiagency teams believed that it appeared to increase their workload and increased the time required with a particular case, hence making this a potentially more costly way of working. It is probably true that to keep different organisations talking together and to provide seamless and timely care for people with complex needs will require a whole new way of thinking about workloads and about information sharing and confidentiality issues. There are a number of differing models of collaborative working put forward in the literature, but they all rely on frequent and honest communication between each of the professionals involved and this, as suggested above, can be time consuming and costly and therefore difficult to achieve, as the professionals involved may well need employment cover whilst they are meeting, even if this is only in an informal manner. One of the difficulties when setting up a joined-up team is not really knowing how it will work, and all participating professions' awareness of this.

At its best collaboration can provide a more holistic view of the target individual and their family, which enables support to be better focused to their particular needs, with better strategic planning of services. At its worst, and without a strong lead professional to coordinate the team, no single organisation has sole responsibility for the intervention, and decision making becomes difficult when too many people are involved, then some highly vulnerable individuals can slip through the net. In this case the open levels of communication can become merely 'talking shops' not able to agree upon a strategy, or perhaps more significantly upon funding, so that support is either not forthcoming or is delayed. Challenges to this manner of working usually start with the intransigence of structures, boundaries and protocols of individual agencies and the professionals working within them.

> These differences manifested themselves in a number of different ways ... different boundaries and authority organisation, different working conditions and expectations, interagency rivalries, different viewpoints and priorities and different working methods and roles.
> (Atkinson et al., 2007, p. 7)

For any form of collaboration to work effectively Atkinson et al. (2007) emphasise the necessity for a mutually agreed and strong professional to lead the collaboration, with clearly defined aims and objectives, and the need to develop a commonly agreed language between all members of the team. Whilst agencies have targets imposed upon them by both national and local authorities, and ring-fenced budgets, making money available for joint activities is difficult, and the concept of pooling budgets can be unpalatable to managers and account holders alike. This could be seen as a 'risky investment', as the funds are no longer under the control of the contributing agency. The amounts available to any form of pool are likely to be varied, and this is exacerbated by the need to involve the voluntary sector in any form of collaboration, where funding is often a major struggle.

Despite the negatives, collaboration between professionals has the potential for enormous benefits to the children and adults with IPDs, but it is clearly a complex matter that requires a considerable investment of time, training, finance and professional willingness to make it work. This is likely to involve a change in culture and attitude from the specialists involved, and this needs to be part of the very early training of the various professionals, embedded within all initial training programmes.

The Special Educational Needs and Disability Act (DfEE, 2001) also set into legislation the requirement for all schools, local authorities and professionals working with children to actively engage with parents and the education of their children. This will mean collaborating and working with voluntary and charitable groups, as well as individual parents. The aim was for parents to be involved in the development of policy documents particularly in relation to special educational needs. It is essential that parent partnership is at the heart of any policy related to children, but particularly to those with IPDs, who can be very challenging at times, so that parents, practitioners, teachers and all support services, work closely together to achieve a positive impact on a child's development (Figure 11.1).

Legislation, non-legislative policies, regulation and practice

At a governmental level there are various pieces of legislation related to education which have been passed through parliament that include provision for equal opportunities; the rights of those with disabilities are all now protected by statute, however, there are no dyslexia laws in the UK, and dyslexia and IPDs often fall under an umbrella of more general special educational needs legislation. At a policy level, local authorities are able to make specific regional regulation, as long as it falls within the legislature of the country. This means that local authorities vary enormously, and how each local authority interprets the legislation can also vary widely, so that individuals living in one part of the country can be subjected to a very different set of regulations to those in another. This potentially has the effect on support and intervention, of a postcode lottery, and with such variation in policy also comes variation in the funding allocation to children with IPDs, as a proportion of the overall education budget. Such differences can impact not only the support received but also initial identification and assessment. For this reason, there are often huge differences between local authorities in the number of children identified, and in receipt of support, and this can influence how much of a priority each authority places on the allocation of funding and support for IPDs.

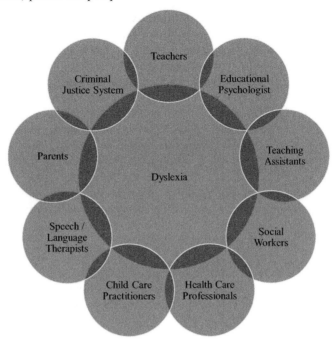

Figure 11.1 Collaboration and the interrelationship with dyslexia

REFLECT ON THIS

Think about a family that you have worked with recently, where IPDs are having an impact.

1 Make a list of the different services that they may have been involved with.
2 What information do you think would be useful for these services to share?
3 What benefits could be achieved for that family of a close working professional partnership?
4 What barriers might impede such communication?

Training

> To establish high quality work in settings and schools requires an investment in training. As training costs amount to a large, if not the largest system-wide investment, the review has considered value for money in terms of the scope and impact of training.
>
> (Rose, 2006, p. 173)

According to Rose (2006), in 2004–2006 the DfES provided around £130 million for training in literacy development. However, Rose (2006) also points out that although there was evidence that the training improved the performance of teachers and practitioners, the training was not always of the highest quality, and he called for improvements to the training to ensure that all who work with young children understand the need to consider the holistic developmental processes that children require, in order to learn to read. This would in turn bring about an urgent need for the upskilling and training of the trainers.

REFLECT ON THIS

Stereotypes of particular professionals will always exist. Consider the stereotypical views of the following professionals, the first one has been started for you:

- Child care practitioners: *Female / young / limited training / poorly paid.*
- Teachers:
- Social workers:
- Health visitors:
- Probation officers:
- Nurses:
- Medical doctors:

How do these stereotypes affect the way that you work with these professionals – this may be positive or negative?

The way forward

When considering the future, we can speculate upon some of the potential changes. Firstly, consider the political culture which will always have implications for policy making, for example, a change in government from left wing to right wing will likely mean an 'all change' environment, as basic ideologies on the purpose and nature of education and employment vary vastly. The move away from the European Union (BREXIT) is already influencing policy making in this field. Secondly, policy cannot be seen in isolation, and will always be dependent upon the bigger economic and political picture, and this has always brought historical tensions and competition, which, in the past, has impeded progress. Thirdly we can speculate upon the ways in which new research, particularly exciting advances in genetics and neuroscience, will influence the precise nature of future government policy.

The way forward clearly needs to include the following ten actions although not in any particular order:

1 The development of a clearly defined and agreed definition, to take account of new research within neuroscience, genetics, education and psychology, to enable undisputable assessments of these conditions to be made, by appropriately trained and qualified practitioners.

2 A series of integrated and coherent nationwide policies need to be developed to ensure that all children, especially those with an IPD, are able to experience an effective pedagogy, regardless of their postcode or socio-economic status. This needs to be research based and take full account of the neurobiology of these children, with an understanding from society that this is a lifelong condition, usually based in genetic origins.
3 More intensive training for all teachers and practitioners, with specialists in the field to support them to adapt their practice, to meet the needs of the children in their care. This will require better trained and knowledgeable trainers, monitored for their practice.
4 Better and more high-quality training, meeting nationally recognised standards, for all childcare practitioners (level 2 and 3), thereby increasing an awareness of their ability to identify very young children and babies who could be at risk of an IPD, in both pre-school and home-based settings.
5 An understanding that the learning differences experienced by these children are not specific to their school years but are lifelong conditions, and young people and adults should be supported beyond school, at pastoral, academic and mental health levels, with policies which allow access to supportive facilities including, individually appropriate assistive technology.
6 Funding that can be allocated according to individual needs, not a postcode lottery of difference between local authorities, and its varying place within their allocation of budgetary hierarchies.
7 Research into IPDs which is enshrined in legislation and consistent across all local authorities, to ensure that all children have an equitable share of support and that all future policy is based on well-founded research.
8 Educational institutions, at all levels, having consistency of policy and practice, ensuring that they are not able to interpret legislation and policy differently to suit their budgetary needs, thereby refusing support on the basis of arbitrary and potentially discriminatory definitions of entitlement.
9 Effective screening and specialist support for IPDs within the early years. This is despite the thinking of Sir Jim Rose (2009), who felt that the blanket screening of all children was inadvisable due to the unreliability of the present screening techniques. He did, however, agree that close monitoring and observation was needed, which required well-trained, knowledgeable and vigilant early years practitioners.
10 More open, transparent and accessible communication between early years settings, schools and other agencies working with children and their families, with an obligation on schools to take seriously their concerns when identifying the children at risk, by continuing to observe and monitor their holistic development, and bringing any concerns to the attention of specialists within the field.

What is really needed is the political desire and wherewithal to commit to fair financial investment allocation, and a societal understanding of the concept of the multiple differences in the way that humans process information in the world. The ten actions for the future, listed above, are certainly not going to be easy to achieve, and there are going to be some significant barriers to success which need to be highlighted before steps to implement them can be achieved.

1. Undoubtably the most significant barrier is going to focus on finance, and concerns of local authorities about the numbers of children who could potentially require support, at a time of huge financial constraint and fiscal restrictions by national government. There is concern about opening the floodgates, which could not be closed in the future. Clearly, as this book has shown, this is a chicken and egg situation, invest early on and rewards will be reaped at a later stage, with increased employment, less dependence upon the benefit system, less strain on health and social services, criminal justice system, etc. However, whilst money is divided into small pots, with those responsible for each pot jealously guarding their right to allocate them, no opportunity for redistribution will exist and no global view can be achieved.
2. There is still no one clear operational definition which society can understand and agree upon. Medical conditions such as measles and chicken pox are clear to define: if you have these observable symptoms you have the disease. Even genetic conditions such as Down's syndrome and cystic fibrosis have clearly defined markers and indicators of their existence in a person. However, IPDs are not diseases, and for the most part those with them do not look outwardly any different from anyone else, making them very difficult to identify. Searching for such markers and indicators must be a priority for future research if these conditions are to be taken seriously.
3. There are currently an insufficient number of trained personnel in the public sector, teachers, prison workers, social workers, health care staff, etc. This will take time, energy and finance to rectify, and needs enthusiastic and suitably qualified trainers to train the staff.
4. There is currently a worrying lack of societal awareness of these conditions, and how they can seriously impact the everyday lives of individuals and their families. A campaign of awareness needs to be implemented.
5. There is currently no clear understanding or agreement of what constitutes an appropriate intervention, which is scientifically validated and research based. This opens the doors to the charlatans and myth makers to make money from vulnerable people, and worryingly the potential to send research into unsuccessful blind alleys, thereby distracting from areas that could really make a difference.
6. The preponderance of investment from 'big business' and commercially driven interventions, which are frequently untested and unsustainable, are perhaps 'muddying' the water, and making it harder for people to know what is reliable and what is not.
7. Screening in the early years is highly controversial, especially the process of agreeing on a method of measurement. A one-size-fits-all method is

unlikely to be effective as it is likely to leave some children and their families abandoned by the political system. When settings and schools are channelled into a particular style of measurement by governments, children with any form of IPD may well feel that they do not 'fit the mould' and schools and teachers view their lack of progress as potentially inhibiting the school's overall progress up the measurement scale, to achieve a higher status and potentially a larger share of the public purse.

8   Inclusion is such a broad area, and IPDs are just one small part. Many people do not have sufficient understanding of what inclusion really looks like and of how, or if, it can be fully achieved or even its desirability.

9   There is currently very poor understanding of what constitutes *reasonable adjustment* and this inhibits employers and those in education, for fear that it will be too expensive or too time consuming.

Conclusion

This book has frequently referred to appropriate intervention, teaching and pedagogy but there is a huge debate to be had about what the most effective provision looks like. What has the most beneficial long-term impact is still highly uncertain, and an area for urgent research. Even the question of whether provision should be fully inclusive, with children attending mainstream settings, or exclusive with children receiving specialist education in delineated schools, or even some form of middle ground system, is controversial. It is, however, apparent that research must lead the way, and that governments of all political persuasions, and at all levels, need to come together behind that research. Unclear and woolly thinking about an agreed definition is impeding progress, and a consensus on causal theory is essential for that. Only with this consensus can key markers be established, to aid identification at an early age without having to wait for failure to occur.

Legislation may be needed in the future to ensure cost-effective methods of lifelong support for individuals in nurseries, schools, colleges and places of employment. This will largely need a cultural change, led by financial considerations. It is possible that this change can only occur when governments and society wake up to the enormous financial drain, across the whole of public services, that IPDs can have, and how society wastes the potential that could be harnessed to enable its progress, if appropriate investment was made in the early years. A book of this sort cannot, and should not, seek to provide answers, but rather in a small way, to pose questions, opening the way for interesting and enlightened discourse on Politics, politics and policy making for the future.

> The total resulting costs to the public purse arising from failure to master basic literacy skills in the primary school years are estimated between £5,000 and £43,000 per individual to the age of 37, and between £5,000 and £64,000 over a lifetime. This works out at a total of £198 million to

£2.5 billion every year, which far exceeds the costs of quality early intervention. At every level, dyslexia and its repercussions are a cause for public concern and an urgent call to action by those responsible for education policy makers and provisions.

(KPMG Foundation: 2006, p. 5)

Further reading

British Dyslexia Association (2019 April) *The Human Cost of Dyslexia: The emotional and psychological impact of poorly supported dyslexia*. https://cdn.bdadyslexia.org.uk/documents/News/May-APPG_for_Dyslexia_and_other_SpLDs_report_-_Human_cost_of_dyslexia_final.pdf?mtime=20190507112230 (accessed 05.05.20.)

British Dyslexia Association (BDA) (2019b, October) Educational Cost of Dyslexia: Financial, Standards and Attainment Cost to Education of Unidentified and Poorly Supported Dyslexia, and a Policy Pathway to End the Educational Cost of Dyslexia. https://cdn.bdadyslexia.org.uk/images/Educational-cost-of-dyslexia-APPG-for-Dyslexia-and-other-SpLDs-October-2019.pdf?mtime=20191024132817 (accessed 05.05.20).

These two reports make for very disturbing and uncomfortable reading, and clearly indicate that the identification and support in the education system of today is far from adequate and that as a society we need to be doing more to harness the talents and support the challenges of those with dyslexia. Both reports were extensively researched by the British Dyslexia Association for submission to the All-Party Parliamentary Group for Dyslexia and other SpLDs. Both reports offer the most up-to-date statistics and information about dyslexia in this country and are essential reading for those who are planning to study this subject in more detail, or to research further IPD in education, the workplace and society in general.

References

Atkinson, M, Jones, M and Lamont, E (2007) *Multiagency Working and Its Implications for Practice: A Review of Literature.* https://www.nfer.ac.uk/publications/mad01/mad01.pdf (accessed 14. 12. 19).

British Dyslexia Association (BDA) (2019a, April) *The Human Cost of Dyslexia: The Emotional and Psychological Impact of Poorly Supported Dyslexia.* https://cdn.bdadyslexia.org.uk/documents/News/MayAPPG_for_Dyslexia_and_other_SpLDs_report_-_Human_cost_of_dyslexia_final.pdf?mtime=20190507112230 (accessed 21. 12. 19).

British Dyslexia Association (BDA) (2019b, October) *Educational Cost of Dyslexia: Financial, Standards and Attainment Cost to Education of Unidentified and Poorly Supported Dyslexia, and a Policy Pathway to End the Educational Cost of Dyslexia.* https://cdn.bdadyslexia.org.uk/images/Educational-cost-of-dyslexia-APPG-for-Dyslexia-and-other-SpLDs-October-2019.pdf?mtime=20191024132817 (accessed 20. 12. 19).

Clough, P (1998) *Managing Inclusive Education.* Sheffield: Sage.

Department for Children, Schools and Families (DfCSF) (2009) *The Common Assessment Framework for Children and Young People: A Guide for Managers.* Leeds: CWDC.

Department for Education (2019) *Participation Rates in Higher Education: Academic Years 2006–2007–2017/2019.* www.assets.publishing.service.gov.uk/government/uploads/

system/uploads/attachment_data/file/834341/HEIPR_publication_2019.pdf (accessed 01. 12. 19).

Department for Education and Science (DES) (1978) *The Warnock Report: Special Educational Needs: Report of the Committee of Enquiry into the Education of Handicapped Children and Young People*. London: HMSO.

Department for Education/Department of Health (2015) *Special Educational Needs and Disability Code of Practice: 0–25*. London: DfE. https://assets.publishing.service.gov.uk/government/uploads/system/uploads/attachment_data/file/398815/SEND_Code_of_Practice_January_2015.pdf (accessed 14. 12. 19).

Department of Health (DoH) (2003) *Every Child Matters*. London: HMSO.

DFEE (2001) *The Special Educational Needs and Disability Act*. www.legislation.gov.uk/ukpga/2001/10/introduction (accessed 14. 12. 19).

Elliott, J and Nicolson, R (2016) *Dyslexia: Developing the Debate*. London: Bloomsbury Publishing.

Henshaw, C (2018) Council attacked for saying dyslexia 'questionable'. *TES*, 31 October.

KPMG Foundation (2006) *Long Term Costs of Literacy Difficulties*. London: KPMG Foundation.

National Literacy Trust (2017) *Adult Literacy*. https://literacytrust.org.uk/parents-and-families/adult-literacy/ (accessed 20. 12. 19).

Nutbrown, C., Clough, P and Atherton, F (2013) *Inclusion in the Early Years*. London: Sage Publications.

Office for National Statistics (2019) www.gov.uk/government/organisations/office-for-national-statistics (accessed 14. 12. 19).

Reid, G (2016) *Dyslexia: A Practitioner's Handbook* (5th edn). Chichester: John Wiley and Sons.

Rose, J (2006) *Independent Review of the Teaching of Early Reading*. London: Department for Education and Skills.

Rose, J (2009) *Identifying and Teaching Children and Young People with Dyslexia and Literacy Difficulties*. Nottingham: DCSF Publications.

Tizard, J (1972) *Children with Specific Reading Difficulties*. London: Department for Education and Science.

Endnote

Firstly, I would like to say a huge thank you to you for choosing to read this book. If you found the ideas contained within it helpful, then please do write a review. It need not be long, just a few words, but it might make others reach for this book and increase the understanding of dyslexia and all its advantages and disadvantages. In turn this may help others with this condition as more people understand how they can help and how they can support those with an information processing difference better.

I would love to hear from you and your comments about the book, both positive and negative, and how you think that writers such as myself, with a passion for this field, can help to spread the word wider in the future. Word of mouth is such a powerful thing, and without you reading books such as this, using them to assist your studies and talking about dyslexia with passion and knowledge, the understanding of this condition in the world outside academia would be very limited.

You can contact me at my e-mail address drcarolhayes@btinterrnet.com

Carol Hayes

Index

Abramson, L.Y. et al. 53, 55
Abuse 28, 59, 64, 82–82, 94, 122
Aetiology 2, 23
Alexander-Passe, N. 35, 38, 60, 61, 62, 65, 72, 94, 108
All Party Parliamentary Group for Dyslexia and other SpLDs (APPG) 51, 55, 121, 124, 189
Alm, J and Anderson, J. 94, 108
Ambitious About Autism 85, 91
Amira, A et al. 55
Anxiety 22, 27, 30, 34, 40, 47, 52, 57, 58, 59, 60–65, 67, 87, 90, 117, 174
Assessment 12, 16, 19, 24, 32, 41–43, 46, 47, 51, 58, 64, 76, 77, 84–85, 88, 89, 96, 106, 116, 117, 166, 183
Association of Directors of Adult Social Services 87, 91
Avramidis, E and Norwich, B. 80, 81, 91

Barriers 10, 36, 49, 76, 78, 102–103, 105, 108, 156, 184, 187
Basic Skills Agency 123, 124
Beetham, J. 116, 124
Behaviour i, 28, 30, 31, 34–35, 40, 41, 47, 50, 51, 53, 60, 64, 79, 80, 83, 85, 87, 93, 94–97, 101, 103, 104, 107, 108, 132, 165, 166, 180
Berryman, M and Wearmouth, J. 49, 55
Bodkin, H. 81, 91
Boyes M et al. 57, 73
British Dyslexia Association (BDA) 9, 20, 49, 79, 89, 101,177, 189
British Psychological Society (BPS) 8, 20
Bullying 33, 35, 92, 97, 113, 170, 171
Burden, R. 37, 38
Burge, B et al. 48, 56
Burns, R. 27, 38

Centre for Studies in Inclusive Education 80, 91
Chapman JW and Tunmer, WE. 30, 38
Cole, EL. 22, 38
Compass 119, 124
Counselling 8, 66, 67, 73
Criminality 91, 93–97, 101–108
Critchley, M. 3, 16, 20, 101, 108
Cultural expectations 47, 50
Cutting, LE et al. 2, 20

Dahle, AE and Knivsberg, A. 58, 73
Dale, C and Aiken, F. 114, 124
Davies, K and Bratt, J. 96, 108
Definition 2–11, 15–17, 19, 75, 76, 90, 97, 116, 128, 133, 158, 178, 185, 187, 188
Delegation 120, 143
Department for Education (DFE) 44, 56, 85, 86, 91, 118, 125, 126, 137, 143, 177
Department of Health (DoH) 44, 56, 79, 91, 116, 125, 126, 137, 143, 177, 181, 190
Depression 26, 54, 56, 59, 63–64, 73, 87
Disclosure 6, 89, 110, 114–116
Donaldson, M. 74, 91
Dore programme 149, 169, 170, 171
Driver Youth Trust 84, 92
Durkheim, E. 101, 108
Dweck, C. 33, 38
Dyslexia Action 84, 92, 95, 101, 108
Dyslexia, Dyspraxia, Attention treatment (DDAT) 169
Dyslexia friendly schools 49, 79, 92

Easton, P et al. 68, 69, 72, 73
Education and Skills Funding Agency 86, 92
Education to workplace 111

Education, Health and Care Plans (EHC) xii, 85–86, 106
Edwards J. 58, 59, 62, 73, 83, 92
Eide, BL and Eide, FF. 111, 125, 127, 132, 134, 135, 142, 143
Einat, T and Einat, A. 94, 108
Elliott, J and Grigorenko, EL. 10, 20, 159, 175
Elliott, J and Nicolson RI. 178, 190
Elmer, N. 58, 59, 73
Employability 102, 110–111, 118
Equality and Human Rights Commission 115, 125

Families viii, x, 17, 11, 37, 40–55, 72, 75, 77, 79, 86, 87, 93, 105, 150, 160, 173, 174, 180, 181, 182, 186, 187, 188
Fawcett, A. 117, 118, 125
Fitzgibbon, G and O'Connor, B. 112, 117, 125
Foss, B. 46, 56
Frith, U. 5, 20
Frustration, resentment and anger 93–94
Funding viii, xiii, 17, 105, 106, 111, 117, 137, 147, 149, 160, 162, 163, 177, 178, 180, 182, 183, 186

Ghouri,, S. 44, 56
Gibb, N. 112, 125
Gough, PB and Hillinger, ML. 15, 20
Growth mindset *33*

Haft, SL et al. 33, 38
Hagan, B. 113, 115, 117, 124, 125
Hampshire, S. 65, 73
Hartas, D. 46, 56
Harter, S. 30, 38
Hawton, K et al. 64, 73
Hayes, C. I, vii–x, 2, 9, 74, 75, 149
Health and care staff 68–71
Heiervang, E et al. 97, 109, 34, 38
Henderson, DA and Thompson, CL. 65, 73
Hewitt-Main, J. 105, 119
Higher Education Statistics Agency (HESA) 5, 20
History **3**, 104, 145, *146,* 177–178
Hoffmann, FJ et al. 115, 125
Home learning environment 7, 46–47, 48
Hunter-Carsch, M. 94, 109

Identification ix, 2, 5, 11, 24–26, 41, 47, 49, 55, 58, 75, 76–77, 84, 100, 106, 107, 130, 139, 147, 155, 158, 183, 188, 189

Inclusion 77–82, 87, 90, 140, 171, 172, 180–181, 188
Inside and out 57–58
International Dyslexia Association (IDA) 8, 9, 20

Kassin, SM. 99, 109
Kirk, J and Reid, G. 93, 94, 101, 105, 118
Klasen, E. 16. 20
Knapp, M et al. 66, 73

Labels 11–14, 15, 24, 107
Lawson, P. 83, 92
Learned helplessness ix, 29–31, 53–54, *104*
Logan, J. 111, 120, 121, 125, 130, 143
Long, R and Hubble, S. 118
Luft, J and Ingham, H. 7

Macdonald, SJ. 101, 102, 103, 108, 109
Mackay, N. 79, 92
Makita, K. 16, 20
Malpas, M. 121, 125
Mentor 105, 106, 121, 132, *138*
Middle-class disease 41–44, 159
Miles, TR. 3, 5, 20
Miles, TR and Miles, E. 16, 20
Miller, JF. 11, 20
Mind 57, 73
MIND strengths 127
Morgan, E and Klein, C. 12, 24, 25, 48, 49, 50, 97, 121
Morgan, P. 2, 20
Morgan, W. 98, 105, 109
Morris D and Turnball, P. 68, 73
Munro, E. 87, 88, 92

Nalavany, BA et al. 88, 92
National Audit Office 66, 73
National Health Service 63, 65, 73, 114
National Institute for Health and Care Excellence (NICE) 66, 73
Newlands, F et al. 68, 73
Nicolson RI and Fawcett, AJ. 11
Non-dyslexic world 36, 54, 72
Nosek, K. 6, 21, 31, 56
Nutbrown, C et al. 91, 92, 180, 190

Office for National Statistics 66, 73, 179, 190

Pacific Centre for Flexible and Open Learning for Development (PACFOLD) 34, 38

Palmer, S et al. 67, 73
Parent Friendly 44–46
Peer group 36, 52–53, 104
Police 23, 24, 96, 98–100, 105
Policy 44, 45, 74–76, 77, 79, 81, 85, 147, 177–189
Poverty 36, *95*, 101, 102, 103, 108, 126, 179
Prevalence viii, 15–16, 19, 68, 76, 78, 91
Prison population 94–98, 105
Psychosomatic disorders 62
Pumfrey, P and Reason, R. 51,56

Qualifications and Curriculum Authority (QCA) 77, 78, 92

Reasonable adjustments 4, 91, 115–120, 124
Reid, G. 7, 9, 19, 20, 47, 48, 56, 59, 73, 75, 76, 79, 92, 179, 180, 181, 190,
Reid, G and Kirk, J. 12, 95, 96, 97
Reliability 150, 160, 161, **164**
Resilience ix, 17, 22, 31, 32–34, 37, 38, 40, 43, 47, 57, 62, 75, 91, 128, **129**, *138*, 179
Retained Reflex Syndrome 169
Rice, M. 97, 109
Rice, M and Brooks, G. 16, 21
Rice, M et al. 97, 109
Riddick, B. 26, 27, 31, 32, 34, 38, 58, 62, 65, 73
Rogers, C. 26, 38
Rooke, M. 34, 37, 38, 131, 143
Rose, J. 4, 8, 21, 184, 186, 190
Rutter, M et al. 34, 38

Saunders, C. 93, 109
Savant Syndrome xiii, 128–130
Scott, R. 64, 73, 81, 82, 86, 92, 115, 125, 128, 129, 143
Self-concept 25, 26–29, 30, 31, 32, 33, 37, 47, *104*
Self-esteem 26–29, 30, *31*, 32, 34, 35, 50, 51, *59,* 63, 77, 88, 90, 91, *95,* 100, 102, 105, 174, 180

Self-harm *63*, 64–65, 66, 97
Self-image 18, 26–29, 50
Seligman, M and Maier, S. 29, 31, 39
Seligman, MEP. 53, 54, 56
Shaw, SCK and Anderson, JL. 35, 68
Shaywitz, S. 45, 47, 56, 64, 73
Sherman, GF and Cowen, CD. 15
Siblings 29, 45, 52, 122
Silver, AA and Hagin, R. 16, 21
Social and emotional consequences 31–32
Social Services 66, 74, 87–90, 177, 187
Socio-economic aspects 7, 41, 103, 104, 108, 162, 167, 179, 181
Spoonful of sugar 58–60
Sroufe, LA et al. 47, 56
Stress 17, 30, 40, 45, 47, 49, 52, 54, 58–70, 83, 98, 113, 116, 117, 149
Suicide *63,* 64, 65–67, 141
Supportive other 104–107

Thomson, M. 60, 73
Timpson, E. 85, 86, 92
Tonnessen, FE. 11, 21
Tsiachristas, A et al. 65, 73

Unnatural act 14–15
Untold secret 46

Validity 150, 161, 162, **164**
Visual Stress 17, 172–173, 149
Vogel, SA and Adelman, PB. 114, 125

Wearmouth, J. 48, 56
West, D. 103, 104, 109
Willcutt, E and Gaffney-Brown, R. 57, 73
Wolf, M. 132, 143, 37

Xia, Z et al. 7, 21

Zone of Proximal Development (ZPD) xiii, 48